Up the Creek with a Paddle

Beat MS and All Autoimmune Disorders with Low Dose Naltrexone (LDN)

Mary Boyle Bradley

Outskirts Press, Inc.
Denver, Colorado

Up the Creek with a Paddle
Beat MS and All Autoimmune Disorders with Low Dose Naltrexone (LDN)
All Rights Reserved.
Copyright © 2009 Mary Boyle Bradley
V3.0

Outskirts Press, Inc.
http://www.outskirtspress.com

ISBN: 978-1-4327-1150-4

Library of Congress Control Number: 2009920234

Outskirts Press and the "OP" logo are trademarks belonging to Outskirts Press, Inc.

PRINTED IN THE UNITED STATES OF AMERICA

Dedicated To Rosemary Konde

It takes a minute to find a special person,
an hour to appreciate them,
a day to love them,
but then an entire life to forget them.

Thanks so much for your time!

"Books are never out of humor or pride,
never envious or jealous,
they answer all questions with readiness,
they teach us how to live,
and how to die;
they dispel melancholy by their mirth,
and amuse by their wit,
they prepare the soul to suffer everything and desire nothing;
they introduce us to ourselves."

Holbrook Jackson

A Special Note from Dr. Bernard Bihari

In 1986, when I first discovered LDN, if I had Mary on my team, this drug would have been approved, marketed and manufactured by a reputable pharmaceutical company. I have no doubt about that.

I have had the pleasure of knowing Mary Bradley and her husband, Noel, for more than six years. Mary's book, *"Up the Creek with a Paddle"*, is a superbly honest and truthful testimony to the benefits of taking Low Dose Naltrexone (LDN). Mary details Noel's success with LDN for his Primary Progressive Multiple Sclerosis in particular, and also includes many other LDN stories from people with a variety of autoimmune diseases.

Mary has been a true soldier and endless fighter in her pursuit to get LDN to the public, so that they too may benefit from taking this once a day, inexpensive capsule and reap the benefits of this amazing drug.

Mary is a gifted author and I am truly blessed that she is in my life, both as a friend and as a valiant crusader on behalf of LDN. She is one of the most passionate and caring human beings that I have come to know.

Bernard Bihari, M.D.
New York City
December 3, 2008

Foreword

Mary Boyle Bradley, in this remarkable memoir, allows you to feel the detailed experiences of her life and that of her husband and family as they tried to cope with the challenges of diseases for which standard medications had no good answers. She involves the reader, in her own inimitable fashion, with her every misstep and triumph as she learns to work with LDN and bring its information to others. As she devotes herself to this important task, Mary Bradley has become one of the most respected advocates for LDN.

As a board-certified specialist in both Internal Medicine and Preventive Medicine for many years, I see LDN to be one of the most significant therapeutic discoveries in fifty years. It is unique in its ability to induce the body to strengthen its own potent anti-disease resource, the immune system. However, every so often, an amazing medical discovery is born that is not the child of industrial R & D or of universities, but is the creation of just one or two individual practitioners - and its fate, inevitably, is to endure many years of rejection by an unbelieving professional medical community.

Such was the sorry experience of two Australian scientists, J. Robin Warren and Barry J. Marshall, for their stunning discovery that most peptic ulcers are really caused by a treatable bacterium which thrives in the stomach's acid.

And such has been the fate of Dr. Bernard Bihari's discovery in 1986 that a low dosage of the pure narcotic-blocker Naltrexone - called Low Dose Naltrexone (LDN) - acts to strengthen the human immune system and thus relieve patients of any further progression from HIV infection or autoimmune disease or even, in many cases, of cancer.

We all hope for new medical breakthroughs to deal with the challenge of such intractable diseases. And we have learned to patiently await those results from any large pharmaceutical company, which appear to be the only available source for the major funds needed to run the costly clinical trials needed to convince the Food and Drug Administration (FDA). Naturally, no such company will choose to study anything that has no patent, thus no promise of profitability.

Naltrexone, at a 50 mg daily dose, was approved by the FDA in the early 1980's for the treatment of heroin abuse, and by now it is many years off patent and is produced as a cheap generic medication. I first heard of LDN in 1986 from Bihari, who has been a friend of mine since childhood. He acquainted me with the impressive results of a clinical study of LDN use he had just run on patients, mainly drug abusers, who had a new disorder that was causing severe infections and had a high mortality (later to be named HIV/AIDS). In comparison with the dismal outcomes of those in the control group, he found that very many of the LDN-treated patients did well. Based on these findings, he went into private practice in order to help treat this new disease, for which there was no available therapy at the time.

In the years since, as Bihari's practice expanded to include patients with a variety of autoimmune disorders and cancers, LDN repeatedly demonstrated a strikingly high level of benefit in comparison to existing treatments. In addition, there have been repeated reports of LDN's positive effects for person's with central nervous system disorders such as Parkinson's Disease, Alzheimer's, motor neuron diseases (such as ALS and PLS) and Autism.

LDN has shown a minimal risk of side-effects and no toxicity. Being a pure narcotic blocker, it is incompatible only with narcotic-containing drugs. All of the observations thus far suggest that its mechanism of action is consistent with the following description:

The low dose of Naltrexone, most often taken by adults as 4.5 mg in capsule form at bedtime, blocks one's opioid receptors for a very few hours (in contrast to FDA-approved Naltrexone 50 mg, which blockades for a full day). These are the same opioid receptors that receive the beta-endorphins (released by the pituitary gland) and metenkephalin (from the adrenal glands). Because of the blockade, the body responds by doubling or tripling its output of endorphins and metenkephalins and, when the brief LDN blockade has ended, these higher levels act to strengthen the immune system, increasing, for example, its levels of beneficial natural killer cells and vital CD4+ cells.

Unfortunately, no pharmaceutical company has yet been persuaded to expend the monies to run the necessary clinical trial in order to gain FDA approval for any of LDN's special uses. It may be that they fear the competition with their existing lines, or perhaps they feel it would be money wasted because the existing generic 50 mg dose would be easy prey for LDN users to buy and dissolve into many small dosages of LDN.

The reaction of patients to LDN treatment has been overwhelmingly positive, but they have been dismayed by the negative reactions received from unbelieving lay persons and most physicians.

With the assistance of my son, Joel, who luckily is a whiz at computer programming, we determined to tell the world about LDN. In 1999, we set up an informational website called www.lowdosenaltrexone.org (or www.ldninfo.org). We have more recently helped organize four annual LDN Conferences, and, to aid discussions, have added an LDN-Yahoo Group (which has grown by this time to over 5,000 members), which one can easily join from the website.

In the hope of achieving general medical acceptance for LDN (which would require FDA approval of its unique claims), it gradually became clear that no number of anecdotal reports could reach that goal. Only a compilation of clinical trial results published in peer-reviewed medical journals might begin to make the powers-that-be attentive to the remarkable LDN story. And, in the past two years, those clinical trials (not one of which was supported by a pharmaceutical company) are finally being brought to fruition, and often by highly rated medical centers. Here is a short list of LDN research accomplishments as of today, but please see www.ldninfo.org for details on all of the research studies:

- A multi-institutional clinical study of LDN for untreatable Primary Progressive MS in which includes endorphin measurements, published in September 2008. Increasing endorphins were measured and only one progression occurred in six months in forty patients!
- A Phase II placebo-controlled clinical trial of LDN

for Crohn's disease at Penn State, expected completion in early 2009. A successful pilot study published in 2007.

- A Phase II placebo-controlled clinical trial on the efficacy of LDN for children and adolescents with Crohn's disease beginning at Penn State.
- A clinical trial of LDN in HIV-infected citizens of - the first scientific study of LDN for HIV/AIDS in Africa -implemented in October 2007, expected to finish in 2009.
- A study of LDN in the treatment of MS at the University of California, San Francisco, implemented in early 2007; positive results reported in 2008.
- A small clinical trial of LDN in the treatment of Fibromyalgia at Stanford Medical Center implemented in October 2007 was positive. Two new larger studies planned, one for adults and one for children with Fibromyalgia.
- An animal research study at Penn State of Naltrexone in a model of a disease that mimics MS, under a small grant from the National MS Society, confirmed the efficacy of LDN.
- Animal research on neurodegeneration at the National Institute of Environmental Health Sciences (NIEHS) suggesting a protective role for Naltrexone.

However, none of the above begins to convey the joy that has been felt by the many thousands of families who thought that hope was lost - until they were able to find LDN and the possibility of returning to a meaningful life with their loved ones.

David Gluck, M.D.
November 16, 2008

Introduction

*"One of the most valuable things we can do for
one another is listen to each other's stories."*
Rebecca Falls

I have a story I want the entire world to hear. I tried to
entice numerous celebrities to help me carry the torch and
firmly believe that one day they will, but right now, they
are not brave enough to take a leap of faith and run with it.
To tell you the truth, I can't blame them because the story
is difficult to believe.

I have been interviewed by various radio stations many
times around Ireland and have spoken at many conferences
in the U.S.. I even tried to get on T.V., but failed. After
each interview and conference, I was happy enough, but
always felt I should have said more. I need a wider audience to understand the whole thing. The story is just so big.
It is my hope that the hero of this story, Dr. Bernard Bihari,

receives full recognition one day. However, in the grand scheme of things, TV, radio and prizes matter very little.

People matter. People really count. Every single person counts and that is why I want to tell my story. I will start at the beginning.

Chapter 1

"It is easier to fake love than to hide it."
Anonymous

I was born in Cook County Hospital in Chicago on June 11th 1971. My parents, Maureen and Vincent Boyle are originally from Arranmore Island off the coast of Donegal, Ireland. I am their fourth child out of five and their only daughter. My three older brothers are named Pat, Phil and Vince and a year separates all of them. There are two years between Vince and me. My parents aptly named me Mary Anne after my maternal Grandmother. Aptly, because even I can see the resemblance.

In many ways I have been blessed with two sets of parents. I rarely say Mom and Dad. Instead, I generally say Mom, Dad, Annie and Neilus. Annie and Neilus Bonner are my Aunt and Uncle, and they live on Arranmore Island, off the northwest coast of Ireland. Neilus is my mom's younger brother and Mom and Annie have always been closer than sisters.

When I was three, Mom and Dad moved back to Ireland and settled in Galway. Their prime incentive for moving home was to educate their family. They had their final child, Kevin, in Galway five years after me, whom we tortured with tales of rescue adoption until he was too old to believe us.

My parents bought Reilly's Hotel in 1976. They renamed it "The Holiday Hotel" because they had their first date in the Holiday Ballroom in Chicago. The nightclub that they added to the hotel, they called "Cheers" for the most part. The Holiday Hotel is situated in the heart of Salthill, two doors down from Seapoint, and it helped rear and educate all five of us.

My parents sold the hotel a few years ago and the house that my dad attached to it, in which we all grew up, has since been demolished. Apartments went up in its place in keeping with the new trend of the area.

Growing up in Ireland I had the best of both worlds because I spent the winters in Galway with Mom, Dad and my brothers, and the summers in Arranmore with Annie and Neilus.

I was educated in Galway by the Dominican nuns in Taylors Hill, and absolutely loved every second. My brothers went to St. Joseph's or the "Bish" as it is known, and they turned out to be keen oarsmen. I played hockey, and clearly remember racing home on my bike after training to beat the six o'clock bells of the Angelus which resounded from the Salthill church.

I graduated from Taylors in 1989 and went to University College Galway (UCG). I had no idea who or what I wanted to be, and even less interest in growing up. I studied Economics, Sociology and Politics. After completing my second year there I decided to go tulip picking in Holland for the summer. My brother, Vince, drove me to Tulla, in County Clare, to sign up, but I was too late because all of the places had been taken. That meant that I would have to work in the hotel for the entire summer of 1991 and I was not happy about that.

Meanwhile, there was a very happy vagabond drifting around the south of Ireland. He was just about out of money, so he decided to stop and have a pint of Guinness in the Holiday Hotel. Mom was working in the bar and they started to talk. His name was Noel Bradley.

Noel was on his fourth year break from his studies in Mechanical Engineering at Jordanstown, outside Belfast. He was originally from Belfast and raised in "the troubles." His parents owned a chain of shoe shops which had been blown up a couple of times, so eventually they decided to get out. They moved to Fahan, on the Donegal side of the Derry border. Noel had recently returned to Ireland after a stint in London, and was delighted to be back on Irish soil.

Salthill is a beautiful seaside resort on the west coast of Ireland. It is basically one long street off a promenade that looks out onto Galway Bay. Many hotels, restaurants and arcades line the street and behind that street, many residential areas are scattered. Noel explained to my mom that he had just asked most of the hotels on the street for work because he was low on cash and decided to stop for a rest before resuming his job hunt.

The Holiday Hotel was comparatively small. It had ten bedrooms, a restaurant, two bars and a nightclub. Like many family businesses, it was too small to pay for enough staff to run itself and give Mom and Dad an easy life. The summer months, however, attracted many tourists to Salthill which meant that extra staff needed to be hired.

As my mother listened to Noel on that day in June

1991, she thought about his poor mother worrying about him and immediately decided to do right by her. Mom fed Noel a home cooked meal and offered him a full time job in the bar starting the following week. She also set him up with very reasonable accommodation and rent in her old house in Riverside.

Noel was a very happy man.

As with every year in the hotel, it took time for the summer team of 1991 to form. It would have been a summer like all others, I am sure, only for my brother, Vince, was hired as night porter. I don't think he was alone for one second of the night shift ever and I am certain that none of us slept very much for the entire summer.

My eldest brother, Pat, was stand in Disc Jockey, and although I tried to be miserable working there, they made it very difficult. I did make a few last ditch attempts to do something else with the summer, but failed. Hence, I was late joining the team. For the evening shift there were two bars, the quiet front and the disco back. For my first shift I landed the back with Noel.

The back bar looked out over a long rectangular dance floor that was surrounded with booths. The walls had mirrors instead of wallpaper to make the room look bigger. I remember introducing myself to Noel. I was glad that the music was loud because I was not in the mood for socializing.

The first thing I noticed about Noel was that he was obviously high on life. He was dancing. The disco back was the fun bar and we had fun working it. I also noticed, with relief, that Noel was a competent barman. Actually, he was a *great* barman. He knew how to make every cocktail to perfection and he was fast. He had all the signs of a natural and I was relieved that he didn't need training.

The music usually stopped at about 1:30 a.m. and we

4

generally had the place cleaned up and ready for the breakfast crew by 3:00 a.m.. That was when Vince would start
the night porter shift. He made it difficult for anyone to go
home by starting some crazy competition or insisting that
we had something important to celebrate. So, we all hung
out a lot that summer in the middle of the night keeping
Vince company.

Vince and Noel became good friends instantly. They
initiated a joint quest for the perfect woman and were most
entertaining. They tried very hard to find the perfect
woman and amazingly, many women were willing to try
out for the title, but as the summer months passed they
couldn't find what they were looking for. Then, the strangest thing happened.

It was our tradition by the end of July to jump into
Galway Bay predawn. One early dawn, we were swimming
in the Bay and Noel kissed me. That was it. He declared to
everyone the following evening that his quest for the perfect woman had ended. We just clicked. We really clicked.
For the rest of the summer we took our days off together
and worked the same shifts. We became inseparable and I
know that some people referred to us as "the painful couple."

Summer was coming quickly to an end and that meant
reality for most. I had another year to complete in UCG.
Late August, Noel asked me to marry him and I said yes.
We needed a plan to decide what to do next, so we made
one. Noel decided that he wanted to go back to Jordanstown, in Belfast, to finish his degree so that he could
get a better job. It would be the following year before he
could do that because he had to reapply to the college. I decided I would study my Masters degree with him in Jordanstown so we could be together. Meanwhile, he could
work in the bars in Galway until I completed my BA in

Galway. That was our plan. It all made perfect sense and we were incredibly happy. I remember feeling so very happy. I will never forget that feeling.

Then, Noel's left foot went to sleep and would not wake up.

Chapter 2

*"We are all in the gutter, but some of
us are looking at the stars."*

Oscar Wilde

It was one of the very last days of August 1991 when Noel came to work earlier than usual and mentioned casually that his left foot felt like it was sleeping for the past couple of days. We all joked about it and told him to slap it around a bit. We told him that it was good that at least part of him was getting some rest. Nobody took it in any way serious.

Summer ended, the team split up, and everyone went their separate ways. I went back to UCG and Noel stayed on working for Mom and Dad in the hotel. He reapplied to Jordanstown to finish his degree as planned and was instantly accepted. He was due to start his final year of Mechanical Engineering in September 1992 as a mature student. He was twenty-five and I was twenty-one.

In order for me to study in Jordanstown I needed a scholarship. To guarantee a scholarship I needed a 1st Class BA, so I worked for it and I got it. I phoned Jordanstown and a lady from their administration staff offered me a European scholarship on the spot. It covered all fees and also included ninety-five pounds sterling a week spending money. That was enough money for Noel and me to live on if we also worked in the student union bar a night or two a week. It was more than we could have hoped for and I was ecstatic. I instantly accepted her offer and she promised that she would forward me all of the documentation that I would need to formally sign.

The Masters offered by Jordanstown was exactly the course I was looking for. I wanted to study Computing and Information Systems so I could actually do something at the end of it, like write a program, or at least turn on a computer. The job market needed such talents and was offering competitive salaries, so I was excited.

I waited everyday of summer 1992 for the written confirmation that was promised. It fast became late summer. I silently noticed that Noel was still slapping his foot around trying to wake it up. A new team had formed and gelled in the hotel. Vince was no longer night porter and Pat was no longer DJ. It was time to move on, but the letter never arrived.

The disaster that followed is one true testament to the fact that everything happens for a reason. I don't believe in coincidence. Early September came and I called Jordanstown to let them know that I never received any written confirmation. They assured me they sent it to me, but because I had not responded in time, they offered my scholarship to somebody else. It was no longer available. I hung up the phone and I was very angry because I knew that something was not quite right.

I ransacked the mail and asked everyone if they had seen a letter from Belfast addressed to me during the summer. Nobody claimed to have seen it.

I went out to the reception area and Mom called me over to the fireplace to talk to me. She looked visibly shaken. Mom told me that she received the letter and burned it. She told me that she was sorry and explained that she panicked. She said that she didn't want me to go to Belfast when I had my choice of universities and scholarships. She explained that it had nothing to do with Noel. She was always very fond of him. She simply didn't want me anywhere near the bombings. I was very angry. I could not understand her actions and I lashed out untamed. Mom was tough, but she cried. I knew that she was sorry, but I could not stop venting.

Noel arrived to work later that evening and I told him what had happened. He didn't consider it a big deal because he understood my mother's concerns. Noel said that he would still finish his degree in Jordanstown and that I could study a Masters in Galway.

I had my heart set on the course in Jordanstown at this stage so I phoned the University again. I asked them if the same scholarship would be available to me the following year. They said they would hold one for me considering the circumstances. I asked them to please do so and decided to take a year out from my studies to travel.

Mom never forgave herself for burning the letter and deeply feared, at the time, that I would never return to my studies. If ever anything bad happens to me now, I always wonder how I will look at it after a few years of hindsight. Looking back now, Mom burning the letter, was the best thing that could possibly have happened to us in the long run. It was that year out that led to a particular chain of events that could never have occurred otherwise.

September 1992 came and Noel started his final year of Engineering at Jordanstown. I planned on touring France, but ended up drifting around Ireland for the year working odd jobs here and there.

By the end of his course, Noel's left leg was sleeping from the knee down. Looking back, you would think that he or I would have addressed the issue by this point. We didn't.

Noel got a job in Belfast with a small company shortly after he graduated, and I started my Masters degree in Computing and Information Systems in September 1993 as our new plan dictated. I remember noticing towards the end of my studies that Noel's balance was very bad after a couple of drinks. Still, I did not address it. I was not able to address it.

I went to the summer job fare in Jordanstown on June 12th 1993, and was offered a job in London with a financial software company called Wilco. It was the only year they ever interviewed in Belfast. Had I completed the course a year earlier I would never have heard of Wilco and to make a long story short I would never have landed in New York and I would never have met Dr. Bihari. If I had moved to the U.S. independently, without Wilco, it would have been Chicago that I would have targeted because I have a lot of family based there still.

Wilco offered me a job on the spot and it was just the job I was looking for, but I was not keen on the idea of moving to London at the time. However, the company Noel was working for went bankrupt and he was out of work and finding it difficult to get another job so money was tight.

We needed a new plan, so we made one. Noel decided that he wanted to do a Masters degree to improve his chances of getting a job. He secured a grant for the Masters

I had just completed and our new plan formed. I would accept the job in London. Noel would complete his Masters and then he would apply to Wilco for work the following year and join me in London.

We did not address his sleepy leg. We could not address it.

Chapter 3

"Some of us think holding on makes us strong;
but sometimes it is letting go."
Herman Hesse

I moved to London in September 1994 and Noel started his Masters in Jordanstown. I was very lucky because my brother Pat was already setup in London. He was working for Dorling Kindersley and living in Clapham Common. He took me under his wing. I loved living with Pat. There are many sides to Pat and he is always interesting and fun to be with. I flew to Belfast regularly to see Noel and we were constantly on the phone to each other.

Early 1995, Noel called me. His left foot was completely numb at this stage and his right foot was starting to go to sleep. He made an appointment at the Royal Hospital in Belfast because it was time to address the issue. The outcome of his appointment still puzzles me.

They did an MRI and told Noel that they didn't think that he had Multiple Sclerosis, but they could not be sure. They said that they look at three things to diagnose MS, namely a clinical evaluation, an MRI, and a lumbar puncture to examine the fluid in the spine. If you show signs of MS in any two of these then you have MS.

Years later we showed his MRI from the Royal to a neurologist in London who could clearly see scarring, indicating that the MRI showed signs of MS. I am surprised that the clinical evaluation in Belfast did not concur and also surprised that they did not do a lumbar puncture. However, it was 1995 and pre all MS medications. There was no treatment, so there was no rush to diagnose because there was nothing to offer.

The doctor left Noel in limbo by saying that there was a good chance that the numbness would go away, but pointed out that it might get worse and if that started to happen, then they would look into it further. So, they basically told Noel to carry on with everything as normal and to hope for the best. I am an expert at hoping for the best, so I was completely elated with the news. Everything was going to be just fine.

Summer 1995 came and Noel opted to complete the dissertation for his Masters in Thessalonica, Greece. I took two weeks off work and joined him there. It was very hot. I clearly remember noticing that if there was a stool available he would always use it.

I did not address it. I could not address it. Everything was going to be just fine.

Noel achieved his Masters with distinction and Wilco offered him a job as we had hoped. He moved to London and started working for Wilco in October 1995. In January 1996, he bought me an engagement ring and we planned our wedding for October 1996. I knew that something was not right, but for the life of me, I could not put my finger on it. I developed severe panic attacks that summer and had to take off work. I jumped on a plane and went home to Galway.

It felt great to be home. There is no place like home. Mom and Dad were so happy so see me and could not do enough. My brother, Phil, was studying medicine, at the time, and it became his turn to take me under his wing. He was working at his desk in his room that he used to share with Pat. It had two twin beds overlooking the Promenade. I loved that view of Galway Bay. I entered and stretched out on Pat's bed and told Phil that I was losing my mind. He was surprised, but happy to see me and asked me to tell him everything. I was as honest as I could be at the time.

I told him that it all started on the tube ride to work one morning. The underground tubes in London during rush hour were packed tight and nobody ever spoke to anybody. I said that I was standing near the exit holding on to a ceiling hand rail when I felt the whole world spin. My heart thumped so loud that it echoed in my head. My breathing became fast and uncontrolled and I broke out into an instant sweat. I told Phil that I thought that I was going to faint. The gut wrenching furnace of fear I felt inside that made me want to sprint for miles was the only thing that prevented me from keeling over. It was absolutely terrifying.

As time passed, these episodes became more frequent so I went to a doctor in Sydenham, London, who referred me to a psychiatrist at the hospital. I was annoyed that he thought the problem was all in my mind, but decided to see the psychiatrist to prove him wrong.

I never did see the psychiatrist. I went for my appointment, but could not wait in the waiting room because there were too many crazies there. There was a guy screaming at a wall, another banging his head off a chair and a lady having a full-scale conversation with herself. She even moved position to answer herself. They were all products of lonely London. All people whom the system had failed. They epitomized everything I hated about London and how it operates. I left. I needed to run.

I called Noel and told him that I was on my way to the airport. I had to get out of London. I had to go home. I also called my manager in Wilco. She was wonderful. She told me not to worry about work and to take as long as I needed.

Phil looked at me and told me that I would be fine. I was shocked at how calm he was. I was also shocked by the speed of his diagnosis. Then I realized that he related far too well to my situation. He told me that I was having panic attacks. He shared with me that my maternal grandmother lived with them most of her life and that he was also prone to them himself. We inherited a tendency to have panic attacks.

I was wired at this stage. I had not slept in days because every time I was about to drift off my heart would start to race and a gripping fear would make me pace the room. I couldn't eat because every time I tried, my stomach would clench with the same invisible fear. I was glad to lose a few pounds before the wedding, but I was very aware that I was losing my strength. Phil gave me valium to knock me out, but initially I didn't want to take it. I wanted to beat the attacks on my own now that I knew I had a mental issue. I asked Phil if he popped valium nightly and he said that he didn't, but he told me that Grandma did. I asked him how he conquered his anxiety and he told me that he prayed Mathew 6; 25-34. I did not understand what he was talking about. I popped a couple of valium and went to my childhood room and slept like a baby. The next morning at breakfast, Phil started to ask me about Noel.

I talked and talked about Noel. I talked about how well

he was doing at work. He was climbing the ladder fast. He was proving to be a computer whiz and he loved his job. I talked about our nights out in the West End and all the friends we made. I talked about how he went out one morning to buy me an engagement ring like he was going out to buy a loaf of bread. I joked that I should never have accepted the ring until he got down on one knee. Getting down on one knee is simply not Noel's style. I talked about everything, but I did not talk about the numbness in his legs. I could not talk about it. I didn't even know that I could not talk about it.

Phil pressed me a little. He specifically asked if Noel's foot ever woke up. I told him that it didn't, but I immediately clarified that it was nothing because he got checked out at the Royal in Belfast and they told him to carry on as normal.

"Thank God it was nothing!" I said.

Phil pressed more. I told him that the numbness had spread a little, but assured him that it was nothing. Then, Phil asked me if Noel had health and life insurance. I laughed and said no. Phil said that it would be a good idea for Noel to get all of his insurance papers in order before going for any more tests because it seemed clear to Phil that Noel had Multiple Sclerosis.

I cracked up laughing.

I asked Phil if he had read the "Good bedside manner" chapter of the "How to be a Doctor" book, and if so he should brush up on it. Phil can be serious. Phil was deadly serious. I told him that he was crazy, but assured him that I appreciated his concern. This time he was just so far off the mark. Noel was fine. The neurologist said so. Everything was going to be just fine. I just had to find a way to stop my panic attacks and get on with my life. I had a party to go to in October. I was getting married.

Noel phoned me every evening after work and that night in late June 1996 I told him that poor Phil suspected that Noel had MS. Noel was calm. He said that if he had MS then he had MS, to him it was not a big deal. He told me that everyone has to play the hand they are dealt in life, and then he asked me if I had sorted my head out.

"No!" I laughed, but then I told him that I was going to head up to Arranmore Island and get to the bottom of it. I explained that I was going to ask Grandma for the cure. Until then I would get by on valium.

Chapter 4

"To the world you may be one person,
but to one person you may be the world."
Josephine Billings

I love Arranmore Island. Annie and Neilus own the island restaurant and it is always my first stop when I get off the ferryboat. There is nobody in the world like my Aunt Annie. She is more than my Aunt. Mom and I agree that Annie is an equal mother to me. Annie is the most fun-loving, generous, young-at-heart and caring person I have ever met. Everybody who has been privileged enough to have visited Annie goes back to see her again and again. She is godmother to me and all of my peers and many others. My goal in life is to be more like Annie. I think about her all the time. Everybody absolutely adores Annie Bonner.

Attached to her restaurant, is a video games room and a

candy counter, and all of the island children gather and play there just like I did with my peers when I was growing up. I laugh every time I visit because I usually get caught at that candy counter. Every family operates differently. I have many memories of falling for the "stand there for five minutes" routine, both in the bar in Galway and the restaurant in Arranmore. After five hours of standing I can still hear my dad laughing and asking me, "Did you learn anything?"

I arrived in Arranmore and dropped my bags in Annie's restaurant. I avoided the candy counter and headed up the bray to Grandma's house on the bridge. Grandma was ninety-five. She was always very strong and insisted that she was never overweight, she was just big-boned with fluid retention. A bird could eat more than her, she claimed. She looked weaker than usual and told me that she was ready to die. I asked her to hang on until the party in October, but she teased that she'd had her fill of weddings and funerals.

I asked her if she ever had panic attacks. She asked me what they were, so I explained, and she understood. She told me that I was blocking something and that I had to figure out the puzzle for myself. She said that it might take years and that indeed I might never get to the bottom of it. Then, I asked her if she took valium. She said that she didn't know the names of all of the pills that she took. She knew exactly the size, color, shape and purpose of each one, just not the names. Nobody could ever give her a placebo. I looked at her supply and told her that she did take valium.

"Mary dear, that is my sleeping pill of many years," she said.

I told her that I didn't want to be on pills for a mental issue and she laughed from her heart. I asked her what she thought I could be blocking and she told me that she hadn't a clue.

"Maybe you have a bad dose of the wedding jitters," she said.

We laughed a lot together. That evening we hung out and drank hot chocolate. It was our last visit together. Grandma died in July that year.

I headed back to Galway and asked Phil to explain how best to deal with the attacks. He gave me a two week supply of valium and told me to pray. I told him that I didn't want to pray.

"Then you better pray to want to pray," he said, "And don't forget Mathew 6;25."

It was time to go back to London.

Noel met me at Heathrow airport. It was obvious at this stage that standing for long periods of time was starting to get very difficult for him. I made a silent mental note. We were so happy to see each other. I was looking forward to going back to work and our wedding was approaching. I had a wedding to organize and Noel had a honeymoon to book. Everything was going to be just fine.

I eased back into work and started to master the panic attacks when the valium ran out. It was difficult, to say the least, but they taught me how to pray.

October came, so we flew to Galway. We had a wonderful wedding. It was the first Boyle wedding. Vince was Noel's best man and gave a comical speech with much reference to their antics when they worked in the hotel together. Everybody had a good time. I distinctly remember the wedding dance with Noel because he stood on my feet three or four times. I had a mild panic attack after the dance, but nobody even noticed because I had a coping mechanism in place at that point. I had mastered them. I used to focus intently on a memorized version of Mathew 6; 25 and they would pass.

I always laugh when I remember our wedding day because towards the end, my brother, Pat, joined the wedding band and made everyone forget about the video and go completely crazy. It is the funniest wedding video I think I have ever seen. It is the video that taught all of us how not to dance at weddings.

After a wonderful honeymoon in Jamaica, Noel and I returned to London and went back to work. A year passed and by then Noel was completely numb from both knees down. We took the Eurostar train to Paris from London for a weekend for our first anniversary, and I remember he had a great deal of trouble with the steps of the Eiffel Tower. I also remember that he found it difficult to stand for a few hours when we were out and if a stool was available he automatically sat.

On occasion, Noel would test himself by running across the park in London for no apparent reason. He never talked about it, and I never asked. I could not ask. It was completely invisible to everyone and very easy to forget about. The panic attacks were a rarity, but they still lingered.

Christmas 1997 came and we found out that I was pregnant. Noel was absolutely over the moon. We both were. We were ecstatic. I had a very healthy pregnancy and insisted that Noel attended the birth. I figured that it couldn't be that bad an experience. I actually thought that he might even enjoy it.

I went into labor on September 2nd 1998 and paged Noel. His mother, Maura, was visiting us, at the time, and we always laugh at how I kicked off the labor. I walked round and round the docks at Surrey Quays refusing to stop until labor started. As soon as I was admitted, Noel arrived at Kings Hospital in London. He had developed foot drop of the left leg, but it was so slight that nobody noticed it and besides, it was only ever apparent when he was under a great deal of stress or overtired. But, it was there.

The labor lasted sixteen hours and the epidural failed. The cord got caught around the neck of the baby and her heartbeat kept dipping very low. Things were tense for a while. At last, Annie Kate arrived, but she was blue and didn't cry, so they took her away to a corner of the room to work on her. Noel very nearly fainted; he went pale and started to sweat. Thank God, Annie Kate turned a healthy pink and started to roar. When Noel's color returned, I remember thinking that he looked like the happiest dad on the planet. He was so proud of his daughter. Annie Kate was purposely named after my Aunt Annie and her mother Kate.

Shortly after Annie Kate was born a close childhood friend of mine, Coirle, visited us in London. She told me that her sister, Alma, married a wonderful guy named Robert Joyce. She shared with me how much in love Robert and Alma were, but added that she was concerned for them both because Robert was diagnosed with Multiple Sclerosis. She described his symptoms as having numb feet. She said that he was wobbly after a couple of drinks and very tired in the evenings. I asked her what exactly MS was. She told me that she didn't really know, but just knew that as MS went, Robert was very lucky. She assured me that Robert had the best possible type of MS. I felt bad for Robert and Alma on hearing the news.

"That is a very tough hand," I said.

I told Coirle that it made me appreciate having a healthy husband and child all the more.

"Good health is everything!" I stated, and Coirle completely agreed.

At this stage, Noel and I were living in a beautiful company apartment in Surrey Quays in London because we were awaiting a transfer to Dublin. Wilco had plans to open an office in Dublin and I was very happy about that. I desperately wanted to raise my family in Ireland. I wanted to be near Mom, Dad, Annie and Neilus, and I felt that I had traveled enough. Things could not have been better. Then came November 1998.

Mom and Annie came to visit us briefly in London to meet Annie Kate. We had a lot of fun together as always and were deadly excited about the upcoming job transfer. Shortly after that visit, Noel had to go on a short business trip to Frankfurt. By the time he returned his symptoms were very pronounced and very visible. The culprit of the panic attacks was about to come out into the open and that is when the real roller coaster took off.

Chapter 5

*"And you will know the truth,
and the truth will set you free."*

John 8:32

Noel came home to our apartment in Surrey Quays one day after work in November 1998 with a staggering gait. He looked like he was about to fall over on every step. He used the walls of the apartment in the halls to get around because the numbness was rapidly spreading up his legs. It was scary to watch, to say the least.

He staggered into the living room and started playing with Annie Kate. Amazingly, he joked and laughed with her as if he didn't have a care in the world. Equally amazingly, I didn't say a thing. I went into the kitchen and started to cook the dinner as usual. As I peeled the potatoes and focused on that short prayer, Noel called into the kitchen from the living room. He said that maybe I should make an appointment with a doctor for him. I agreed and continued to prepare our meal and he continued to play with our baby.

I never did take Phil's advice regarding insurance so we didn't have private health insurance which meant we were reliant on the National Health Service (NHS) in London. We went to a doctor in Surrey Quays and he told us that Noel had to see a neurologist. The waiting list to see a neurologist on the NHS, at the time, was about eight months. That was too long for us to wait so we decided to go private and pay in full. We met with one of the top neurologists in London. He reviewed the MRI from the Royal in Belfast, performed a series of cognitive tests, did a lumbar puncture and took a very detailed health history.

I will never forget going in for the results. We entered his office and he asked us to sit down. Noel was holding Annie Kate. The neurologist looked happy and said that he was incredibly relieved because initially he was convinced that Noel had a brain tumor. He said that there was no brain tumor and qualified his excitement with that fact that Noel had Multiple Sclerosis. I broke down. I had a complete meltdown. Noel was calm.

"Shit happens," he said.

That is all he said.

I calmed down, realizing immediately that I needed to know absolutely everything. The neurologist said that Noel had Primary Progressive MS and that he would keep getting worse and worse over time. He said that he could not give us a timeline of progression and explained that with MS, each person is different. He wasn't certain if Noel's MS would progress slowly or quickly, but he was certain that Noel's MS would progress.

Noel asked if Annie Kate was at risk of contracting MS and the neurologist assured him that as far as he knew, she was safe, but added that Noel's siblings had a higher risk than normal of developing the disease. I asked the neurologist what we could do to fix it. I asked what medication was available. He replied that there was nothing we could do to fix it and assured me that there were no medications to help Noel. On hearing that I really lost control.

"How could there be *nothing*?" I yelled.

The neurologist said that if Noel had the Relapsing Remitting form of MS, there were various beta interferon medications, but for Noel there was nothing because he had Primary Progressive MS. I felt that the diagnosis was worse than a brain tumor at the beginning because there was no operation to at least try to fix it all.

Noel thanked the neurologist and we left. I was a mess. I was a complete mess. Noel told me to cheer up.

"It could be worse," Noel said.

"How so?" I asked, "What on earth could be worse?"

"You could have it," he said.

"But why do you have it," I said, "Why you?"

"'Why not me?" he replied.

That night, after Noel put Annie Kate to sleep, he stumbled into the living room and found me crying. I found his diagnosis very difficult to accept. I asked him how could he be so calm about it all. I desperately wondered what was going on in his mind. He sat down and told me that he would share his secret. He told me that nothing could bring him down ever again and he would tell me why. I knew his life history, but never knew his real perception of it all.

Noel told me that when he was growing up in Belfast, the lack of respect for human life always deeply saddened him. He had a pretty lonely childhood. Then, when he went to boarding school in Newry, there was an alcoholic priest, Fr Finnegan, who inappropriately fondled many of the young boys in his trust. Noel was one of his victims. That experience set Noel on a course of self-destruction. When Noel entered Jordanstown the first time, he was spiraling downhill. He left his studies and tried to escape in London. There, he worked in some building sites and many bars and became deeply depressed. Eventually, he tried to end his life by jumping off a building. He hit rock bottom. He still questions if that fall triggered his MS. Maybe there is a connection, but it doesn't matter. Shortly after surviving that experience Noel figured everything out. I suppose you could say that he had an epiphany.

Noel woke up one morning and saw God in everything. Every living thing suddenly mattered to him. He came to see himself as just a small part of a wonderful creation and he became very grateful for every breath. He developed a huge appreciation for life. He suddenly saw the beauty in everyone, every single person. He gained a new respect for the gift of life. He forgave Fr Finnegan. He came to believe that the priest was lost and deserved help.

That night, Noel told me that no matter what life threw at him, he would be able to handle it. Obstacles must be expected, he insisted. They are a part of life. Necessary even. Noel was determined to live right, as part of a bigger beautiful creation, as if he had a test to pass, a role to fill or a part to play. If he had one day, two or ten left to live, he was determined to make the most of every second and to keep going and going until he could not go any more. It was that simple. He said that he could deal with having MS because he was alive. In his mind, he had suffered worse. Noel told me that he had never been happier than then because he had a wife and a child whom he loved with his heart and soul, and such love was all that mattered. He thought himself so much luckier than most.

"Believe me Mary, MS is not a big deal." Then, he hugged me.

That day marked the last of all of my panic attacks. They were firmly put to rest.

Chapter 6

"To believe that God never gives us more
than we can handle, one must believe
He wants us to let Him handle everything."
                                        Mary Bradley

I was looking forward to our transfer to Dublin. We would have a great deal of family support in Ireland. Then, something happened in the stock market in Tokyo in late 1998, and the effect rippled across all of the stock markets. A Wilco office in Dublin was no longer a viable option and that meant there was to be no transfer home.

It was coming up to Christmas 1998 and my brother Vince was getting married, so we decided to fly home for the wedding. Just before we left, Noel was offered a job transfer to New York. Wilco wanted him to start in January 1999. We decided to discuss it over the holidays. I was tired and Noel's gait was unbalanced, to say the least, but we were happy. We truly were happy. We were a family.

We arrived home, and as always it was great to be home. Vince was delighted to have found his perfect woman, Helen. I set them up some years prior. Helen studied with me at UCG and I knew that she would be the perfect woman for Vince. Vince is a wonderful guy. My four brothers are great guys and I don't think I am being biased in saying that because anybody who knows them would agree. I think they are brilliant in everything they do.

The wedding party gathered in Galway and the celebrations started. Everybody was obviously and naturally shocked by the decline in Noel. They didn't know what to do or say, so everybody ignored it. We all carried on as normal. We sat in the living room with the large windows looking over Galway Bay and told funny stories. Annie Kate was the star attraction. Everybody loved her instantly.

Later that night, I headed out to catch up with an old friend who was just back from the U.S.. She was home for the christening of her first child. I called out to her house and her sister was there. Her sister was a physiotherapist in London, so I told her about Noel. She told me that in her experience and knowledge, Noel had five more years left to live. She told me that nobody ever tells patients with Primary Progressive MS the truth, but assured me that within five years Noel would be bedridden with feeding tubes. Dead even, or wishing he was. I couldn't take it in. I left.

Thank God, Annie and Neilus were staying with Mom and Dad for the wedding. I arrived home and signaled Mom and Annie from the living room. I told them what I heard and broke down again. Annie told me that she knew people with MS who lived to be a ripe old age. Mom told me that she was going to visit the Poor Clare Nuns in the morning and that everything would be just fine.

"God never gives you more than you can handle," she said.

I told Mom and Annie that I was not going to make Vince's wedding because I couldn't. I didn't want to wreck it on them. Equally, I did not want Noel to realize my true messed up mental state. I desperately wanted to be strong and happy for him, so I instructed Mom and Annie that it was their job to cover for me by whatever means necessary. I needed time, so I went to bed early with Annie Kate and an apparent headache. It felt good to have Mom and Annie support me and I slept well.

The next day, Mom went to visit the Poor Clares. The Poor Clares are a community of nuns who have been in Galway since 1642. Their vowed life of poverty, chastity and obedience is lived in enclosure. It is common practice in Galway to ask these women to pray for special intentions. Their monastery is based in Nuns Island. The Poor Clares gave Mom the name of a doctor in Cork, Dr. Muriel. They told Mom that Dr. Muriel had Primary Progressive MS and asked them to give her number to anyone in need of MS counseling. Mom, Annie and I went to the reception area of the hotel for privacy and dialed the number.

I feared it was going to be a difficult phone call. I felt dreadful that this woman had this disease and had no idea how to ask her how long she had left to live, much less her present quality of life. I had no idea when the number was handed into the Poor Clares and, in my mind, I honestly questioned if she was still alive.

Thankfully, Dr. Muriel answered the phone. I introduced myself and told her that my husband was just diagnosed with progressive MS. I explained that my mom got her number from the Poor Clares in Galway, and then I asked her if she was willing to share her story. She was wonderful. She gave me all the strength I needed to go to

Vince and Helen's wedding. She told me that she had Primary Progressive MS for twenty-five years and that she was still self sufficient. She said that she had to give up her medical practice, but assured me that she thoroughly enjoyed life despite a walker and wheelchair. She told me not to give up. She gave me hope. When I hung up, Mom, Annie and I were so relieved. Dr. Muriel was a Godsend.

The next day, Dec 28th 1998, Vince and Helen got married. It was a beautiful wedding and everyone enjoyed it. Helen knows how to do things just right and we all knew how to behave for the video.

Afterwards, Noel and I told everyone that we were going to move to New York. Noel was so set on the idea that I didn't have the heart to stop him. I dreaded it. Yet, in my mind, he only had a few more years of quality living left, so I figured that he might as well travel the world when he still could. I decided that I didn't have a great need to settle until Annie Kate started school and that was a long time off. Also, the company only offered Noel a one year contract, so I thought I would be back in Ireland before I knew it. Furthermore, I was still on maternity leave and I did not want to leave Annie Kate for a second. I didn't want to go back to work and the salary increase Noel was promised upon his transfer would make it easier for me to stay at home. I tried to look at the transfer as an adventure filled with stories that I could share.

My family was tactfully deeply concerned. Vince begged me in private not to go. He desperately wanted to help us out. He wanted to be there for us. He wanted us near him. Vince is the worrier of the family and the last to be told anything. He was the child who hung out on the windowsill of Mom and Dad's bedroom if ever they went out for an evening, which was a rarity. I remember he used to run into my room to wake me to tell me everything was okay when they arrived home safely.

Noel's family also came to Galway that Christmas and could not believe that we were thinking of moving to New York, but like the rest they put on a brave face and wished us the best.

Early January 1999, we flew back to London and started to prepare for the transfer to New York. Noel's legs were completely numb, but still strong at this stage. His plan was to work on walking again with the new lack of sensation over the next few months.

Chapter 7

"There is only one happiness in life, to love and be loved."
George Burns

That January, Noel flew to New York a week ahead of Annie Kate and me to sort out our accommodation. A U.S. Company, Automatic Data Processing (ADP) bought Wilco a few years earlier. That meant that all of the benefits for ADP employees were automatically made available to Wilco employees without a medical exam on transferring to the U.S.. Noel was offered all ADP company benefits, so he maxed out on health and life insurance.

We settled into a company apartment on Monroe Street in Hoboken. It was about ten blocks from the Path train that Noel needed to use to get to work. It snowed a lot that January and he fell quite a few times walking that distance. To be honest, I have no idea how he walked that far in the snow, at the time, without breaking his neck. I bought him an umbrella that could double as a cane, but he wouldn't use it.

I visited Hoboken years before through work and I loved it. It is a trendy area with cozy bars and restaurants and convenient for people who work in New York City. This time I didn't like it because it was not baby friendly. Our second floor apartment was in a building with no elevator and had windows that wouldn't open. I hated that. It was quite a workout coming and going from the apartment with all of the baby gear. I also hated that. Annie Kate had the best stroller, but the weight of it was never taken into consideration when I bought it. Also, we didn't have a car. Again I hated that. But what I hated most of all was watching Noel drag himself up the stairs in the evening after work.

Despite all of that we were happy. We honestly were. I was very tired, but happy overall. Noel was unsteady, but he never complained about it. He was still high on life. I admit there were times when I broke down on my own and cried, but I vowed that Noel would never see me cry. I was determined to be strong for him and I knew that I was getting stronger day by day. I could feel it. I really started to toughen up.

About two weeks after we settled into Hoboken I found out why I was so tired. I was pregnant again. Noel was once again over the moon. I was delighted also because I wanted Annie Kate to have a close sibling. I didn't want her to be an only child. My pregnancy confirmed my decision that it was time to find a better place to live and make the most of our year in America. There was no way that I was going to bring a second baby home to our apartment in Hoboken.

I didn't know anybody in Hoboken. I didn't want to know anybody. One morning, after Noel went to work, I headed to the train station with Annie Kate and bought a map. Then I took a train timetable and went home to study it. I came up with a plan. Every morning I would go to the station after Noel went to work and visit each town, one by one, on the Bergen Line until I found one I liked. I had to keep in mind that Noel had to commute this distance on top of his current commute, so I was hoping to find a nearby town that was baby friendly and had a furnished house to rent beside the train station with windows that opened. So, every morning Annie Kate and I searched. It took a while.

Then, one cold, clear morning the train stopped at Ridgewood, New Jersey. I didn't only like it, I loved it. It was beautiful and exceptionally clean. It was spacious yet quaint. It was perfect.

We moved to Ridgewood in February 1999 and settled into 237 Godwin Avenue. It was a three family home and we rented the upstairs section. The house was near the station and every window opened. Without question, Ridgewood was baby friendly and I felt a new lease of life. Noel walked to and from the station every morning and evening. Although he never regained any sensation back in his legs, he succeeded in teaching himself how to walk again.

I was determined for Noel to visit another neurologist. To find the best one I figured that I needed a car. To get a car, I needed a U.S. license, and to get a U.S. license, I needed to convert my London license, and to convert my London license, I needed to do a written test. Shortly after we moved to Ridgewood, we met the elderly couple living in the downstairs section of 237 Godwin. They were Marge and Joe Lawler, from a neighboring town. Their house burnt down and it was in the process of being rebuilt. Marge and I became instant friends. She was a retired school teacher. She didn't have an easy life by any means. She had two sons, and one died when he was twenty-six.

He was the picture of health, but choked on a piece of meat and died. It was a sudden tragedy that most people would probably never overcome, but Marge did. Also, her husband, Joe, was battling with Rheumatoid Arthritis and in bad shape. Despite all of that, Marge was happy. She radiated an addictive, almost contagious, gentle inner peace that I loved. She had a special glow. When I was with Marge, I never doubted that God was real. I could see Him in her.

Marge took me under her wing and helped me settle in. I got my license with Annie Kate on my knee for the written test. They took one look at me and waived the practical Part (the actual driving part) and I didn't blame them. I bought a car, a blue Buick Century 1991. It was from the Buick dealer near the train station in Ridgewood, on Broad Street. The salesman asked me to take it for a test drive, but I told him there was no need because it looked fine. I never drove an automatic before and I was afraid that I would crash it. I paid him five grand in cash and he gave me the keys.

It was a nervous ride home and Annie Kate screamed the whole way. But at last we had a car. Marge laughed at the story of purchase and then taught me how to drive on the highways and around the town. Noel could not drive the Buick. He could not feel the pedals properly with his feet.

As soon as I had transport, I started to investigate neurologists. I firmly believed that if anywhere could treat Noel, it was America.

I started with the phone book because I didn't have access to a computer. I was not familiar with the area so I called every neurologist in the book to see if they accepted our insurance and asked what the wait time for an appointment was. When I had narrowed the selection, I drove by certain offices and ran in to get literature from their office to get a feel of their qualifications, history, specialties and patient numbers. None of them had much information, to be honest. Some told me about the standard medications for MS, but it became very clear, very fast, that America did not know of a cure.

I finally settled for a local group of neurologists. I called and made an appointment for Noel for July 8th 1999. When I told Noel, he insisted that he did not want to go for the appointment. He tried to explain that he did not want to make MS the focus of his life. He figured that the neurologist in London knew his stuff and that we had to accept it. It seemed completely futile to him, he told me, to keep asking every doctor the same questions until I found one who would tell me what I wanted to hear. I told him that I just wanted a second opinion. I wanted to fight. He didn't.

I persisted and Noel finally gave in to humor me. He told me that I made his quest for an easy life very difficult. He eventually agreed that it was probably a good idea to have a neurologist in the U.S., so we went for the appointment.

I really liked Noel's new neurologist. He was very professional. He explained his impressive credentials and told us about all the meetings he attended with the MS experts of the world to keep him up to date with all the latest on MS research. He was the MS expert and I felt safe. He told Noel to start on Avonex, a weekly injection. It would most certainly slow the progression of his MS we were told. I felt so good leaving his office. At last we were doing something to fight back. Noel was calm and willing to give the shots a try.

Noel started Avonex therapy in July 1999. Avonex shots are intra muscular so the needle is about an inch long. They are referred to as beta interferon shots. That means they suppress the immune system because it is widely believed that

MS is the result of an overactive immune system. Clinical studies show that Avonex reduces the relapse rate in 35% of patients with MS. They do not stop the progression of MS or claim to. They slow it down for the lucky ones. I am sure that the neurologist explained all of that, but all I heard was that Avonex slows the progression of MS. I found out much later that Biogen, the makers of Avonex, state that it only works on Relapsing Remitting MS. It is not recommended for Primary Progressive MS, but it was the neurologist's belief (which I appreciated so much at the time) that it was much better to do something instead of nothing. I had no idea what the actual odds of it working were. I knew nothing about the drug other than it was going to work. To keep me optimistic, Biogen sent us monthly newsletters filled with happy people with MS on Avonex.

I offered to administer Noel's shots and he accepted. We picked Saturday night because we were told that he would suffer flu like symptoms for a day or so after the needle for up to nine months. I remember the first shot. Noel mixed it while Annie Kate was kicking on the floor in the living room in Godwin Avenue. My bump was also kicking. I read the pamphlet about ten times. It sounded simple. I had to stick it in his thigh muscle. He handed me the needle and I stuck it in, released the shot and pulled it out. I pressed gently on the injection site with a cloth that came as part of the kit and there was very little blood. It seemed easy enough, but I was relieved to get it over with. That time he didn't feel it.

Every Saturday, we alternated between his thighs although we could have used other muscles. There were times when I hit a vein and his blood spat everywhere and other times I hit a nerve or something and he'd jump his own height. It was always a relief to get the shot over with, but as time went on it became part of our routine. I remember one beautiful Saturday morning we went to Point Pleasant, on the Jersey Shore. We stayed at the beach all day and then tried to book in somewhere for the night. The only room that was available was in a sleazy motel with a red flashing neon light. Annie Kate fell asleep so Noel measured the shot using the neon light. I remember thinking that it was very funny. When Annie Kate started to talk she was fascinated with the procedure so we put her in charge of the band-aid.

Initially, the flu-like symptoms were very severe. Noel was feverish every Sunday for about a year, but it didn't bother his spirits. He handled it very well. Tylenol and Advil pain relievers became a necessity and as time went on he needed them less and less. The mental relief because we were actually doing something was huge to mc. Our lives were busy so we didn't think about MS too much. Although busy, we were about to get even busier.

Chapter 8

*"Friends are people who know the song in your heart and
can sing it back when you forget the words."*

Anonymous

September 25th 1999, I gave birth to Aisling. I didn't
want Noel to attend the birth because I had learned
that stress was not a good thing for MS. He also needed to
stay home to look after Annie Kate. Mom, Dad, Annie and
Neilus were visiting at the time, so Mom and Annie went to
the hospital with me.

When Aisling was born, Annie Kate had just turned
one, but she didn't walk until she was fourteen months. So,
when the gang went back to Ireland and Noel returned to
work I had very little time to obsess about his MS. Life
took over. I also felt that we were doing all we could to
combat his MS, so I was pretty relaxed about it all. I trusted
Noel's neurologist completely. I loved my girls and I was

very happy. Once again, things were very good and they were about to get a great deal better.

Marge and I spent many hours together debating life. One day, when we were sorting out the problems of the world, she told me that I should join the Moms Group at Nativity Church in Midland Park. I told her that if ever we were organized enough on a Sunday morning we attended mass at Mount Carmel in Ridgewood. That was a rarity, but I knew a couple of people at this point and I didn't feel the need to branch out. Aisling was christened in Mount Carmel. Marge told me that I would absolutely love Nativity. She explained that it was a smaller community with many stay-at-home moms.

"Every stay-at-home mom needs girlfriends," she said, "Nativity is not fancy Mary, it is very simple."

I didn't feel like I needed anyone because I was perfectly content hanging out with my girls and they kept me busy. However, I am sure that it was Marge who left the Nativity bulletin in my mailbox one morning in late November 1999. It read that the Moms Group met on Wednesday mornings at 9:30 a.m. at the church with their children and drank coffee. I decided to take Marge's advice and check it out.

I always laugh when I remember this. I arrived at Nativity with a diaper bag around my neck, Annie Kate in one arm and Aisling in her car seat in my other arm. That was my normality. The room where the moms gathered was upstairs so I had to climb a flight of stairs and was breathless by the time I got to the door. I walked in. It was a huge, plain, rectangular room. The smell of crayons, plastic and old books reminded me of the convent in Ireland. There was a group of women sitting around laughing, most of whom were holding young babies. It was noisy because boisterous toddlers were running around playing happily.

One of the women came over to me and introduced herself as Tia Patterson. She was in the middle of telling a funny story to the group, so as she was saying "hi" she was also turning her head back to the gang to finish her story. As if she knew me all of my life she took my children and told me to sit down.

I sat and she gave me a coffee and told me to relax for a couple of hours. I couldn't believe it. It was the best morning I'd had in years. I felt completely at home and loved all of the women instantly. We bonded like teenagers and as time went on we often reverted to behaving as such. Rain, hail or shine I never missed Wednesday mornings at Nativity for the next while. Of course, I had no idea, at the time, how much I would rely on the women from Nativity in the future.

At that time, Noel's job was going very well. One day, in early December, he came home late and told me that ADP wanted him to stay in America for longer. Noel explained that he loved America. He also understood my desire to live in Ireland, so he decided that I should make the decision as to whether or not we should stay. I told him that I liked America too. I didn't want to move back to London, and I figured that if we moved back to Ireland I would have to go back to work because he would not get the salary in Ireland to support us. I didn't want to put the girls in daycare when I had the option to stay at home with them. I also figured that even if Noel did get a salary in Ireland to support us, I would never find a network of stay-at-home moms like the group from Nativity because most young mothers in Ireland today have to work to raise their families. Another bonus about the U.S. was that I believed that Noel was getting the best medical care possible. It made no sense, in my mind, to rock the boat.

I told Noel that I wanted to stay. Our lease in Ridgewood was due to expire in February 2000, so we decided to go house hunting.

At this stage, Noel's MS was very visible to everybody in the evenings and it was still progressing. His MS progression always just crept up on us. It was so slow that I used to only notice a decline when organizing my photo album.

Soon Noel began to find the forty minute train journey home difficult if he didn't get a seat. Soon after that, I started picking him up from the train station with the girls to make it easier for him because his legs started to get very tired and heavy at the end of the day. I could instantly tell by his gait when he came off the train whether or not he'd had a seat for the journey. I told him that he should get a cane so that people would know that he needed help, but he refused.

When his walk became very bad, which it did at times, he would visit his neurologist and his neurologist would give him steroids. Noel loved steroids. They made him feel great. But, their effect was always short lived. Still, we were very busy and very happy and about to buy our first house. We didn't have time to dwell on his MS.

I went to playgroup one Wednesday as usual and mentioned to the Moms Group that we were looking to buy a house. One of the mothers was a realtor and told me that a house near her was on the market. She said that her best friend grew up in it and that it was reasonably priced. Noel and I went to check it out and instantly put down a deposit. We moved into Millington Drive on March 1st 2000 and immediately added a dormer with the help of the realtor's husband.

For the longest time our only piece of furniture was a three piece sectional. It consisted of a pullout bed that we used nightly, and two recliners with a small table. We also had two cribs. One in the living room for Aisling and one in the back room for Annie Kate. The upstairs was sealed off and the workmen arrived every morning at 8:00 a.m. sharp to work on the dormer. For seven weeks the girls slept through some serious banging and if they couldn't sleep we all hung out at Tia's house. I had to wake the girls up every morning to drive Noel to the station for 7:30 a.m.. We also picked him up every evening at 7:00 p.m..

One morning in spring, as we were heading to the car I felt nauseous. Noel and I looked at each other and laughed. That evening I confirmed that I was pregnant again. As always, Noel was absolutely over the moon. I was also very happy. I had a new outlook on life. It became very important to me that we did everything we possibly could when we were still able. I refused to take one day for granted. We were lucky because Annie Kate and Aisling were very easy babies so I was positive that we could more than handle a third.

The morning sickness persisted and looking back we were comical. The workmen must have thought we were crazy. Noel and I never mastered the art of curtailing our feelings in public. If we are happy, we are happy and if we are not, then we are simply not. One morning, Noel had an important meeting to attend at his office. He loaded the children into the car and was ready to go, but I was throwing up in the bathroom. I couldn't stop throwing up. Noel was getting impatient and yelled from the door for me to hurry up. I went crazy just as the workmen were arriving. I asked them all if they knew of a way to speed up morning sickness. They said nothing. The anger seemed to settle me so we headed to the car. Noel and I were laughing within seconds, but it was around that time he decided to get hand controls for the car and retake his driving test.

During my third pregnancy I remember going for my twenty week scan. The scan revealed two pointers for

Down Syndrome. I panicked because I didn't want the girls to have to deal with any more. I also debated whether or not to tell Noel because I didn't want to stress him out. Noel, however, knows me very well and I can never hide anything from him so I ended up telling him. He told me that if the baby had Downs then it had Downs.

"Downs is not that big a deal," he said.

He truly was not bothered at all. He was obviously still high on life and I decided to join him. I remember feeling, at that time, that we would have handled a baby with Down Syndrome just fine.

Mom, Dad, Annie and Neilus arrived in early December 2000 to welcome our new baby. Mom and Annie, like all Irish women who visit us went shopping. They all go crazy shopping, like really crazy, especially since the Euro was introduced. When I went into labor, Mom and Annie were at the Garden State Plaza Mall. They managed to find a taxi, but the driver had very little English and the pair had very little idea how to get home. All they knew was to make a left at the house with the reindeer. That was their marker. However, every second house had reindeer on their front lawn so they spent hours in that taxi. Fortunately, Noel could drive at this point so he drove me to the hospital and decided to attend the birth. This time, Noel wanted to be there and thank God, the birth was very easy. Sara was born on December 13th and I felt a huge sense of relief when I first held her. She was perfect. That was a special moment.

When Sara arrived, I was happy with life. I was delighted to have three healthy babies. They were an absolute joy. Noel used to rush home from work every evening to be with all of us. At this stage his MS was visible all the time because he had developed obvious foot drop and everywhere we went it was much easier for him if he was pushing the stroller. Also, his bladder was starting to weaken.

His MS was still progressing, but we were happy, busy and high on life. If he dipped a lot, he took steroids and every Saturday I gave him the Avonex shot. We were doing all that we could to fight back. Then two things happened. He got a cane and I got a computer.

Chapter 9

"One word frees us of all the weight
and pain of life and that word is love."

Sophocles

We rang in 2001 with no knowledge that it would prove to be a very difficult year. It is that year that makes me appreciate the good times all the more. In January 2001, Noel bought his first walking cane. Initially it was to help him get to the car in the snow. We bought the cane from Town and Country Pharmacy in Ridgewood. I remember that because of the wonderful service they provided. It was a classy cane. It was black with a silver handle and I was relieved that Noel finally had a cane to help him. I told people that he didn't get it because he progressed. I insisted that he should have had it years ago to make life easier. It is clear, looking back, that he got the cane because he had progressed.

Normally, at that time, when he came home from work in the evenings he would put his cane in the closet. He did not need it around the house initially.

Then in June 2001, my uncle Neilus was diagnosed with Parkinson's Disease (PD). My family and I were back and forth with e-mail all the time at this point. Neilus had a shake in his right arm for some time and although everybody hoped and prayed for the best, we were somewhat prepared for bad news. However, the diagnosis was a devastating blow to all of us. It was difficult to believe that Neilus could have Parkinson's because nobody in our family ever had Parkinson's and Neilus always epitomized masculine strength, so it just didn't seem right.

Once we confirmed that the diagnosis was correct we had to accept it. I have observed a common thread, not only in my family, but also in my dealings with many others. It seems to me that the knee jerk response of people when they hear that a loved one is diagnosed with something like Parkinson's or MS, is to firmly and instantly decide that the loved one has the best possible MS or the best possible Parkinson's. This is easy to do because there is no map to guide anyone through a linear progression. It was a great relief to me, at the time, to hear and believe that Neilus had the best possible Parkinson's. As Parkinson's Disease went Neilus was going to have it very easy. I thought about Neilus all the time that summer and planned a trip home with my girls to be with him.

After my trip home, Mom phoned me to tell me that she found a lump in her breast and her doctor wanted to remove it for biopsy. She didn't want to mention it when I was home in case it ruined my visit. In September 2001, Mom called me to tell me that she had breast cancer.

She was dreading telling me because I was so far away and we are very close. She and Annie feared that my panic attacks would return. I had learned much about life at this point. Phil's tip to pray served me well. I became Mom's support and told her that we were going to beat it together. I assured her that everything would be just fine.

Then, October 2001 came and a very close friend of mine, Paula Lein, from the Moms Group at Nativity, told me that she was recently diagnosed with MS. Fortunately for all concerned, it was the best possible MS you could hope for. As MS went, she was going to have it very easy. My friend was thirty at the time. She had two young children and a husband whose attentive nature landed many of the other husbands from the group in much trouble over the years.

When I was growing up, my dad always told me if ever I was down or just plain old angry that I wasn't looking at things right. He used to say that there is good in everything if you look at it right. I now know what he meant. There *is* much good in everything if you look at it right. For example, I would not wish the good fortune of MS on anyone, but I can clearly see all the good that Noel's MS has brought to our family. It has revealed strengths and attributes that he possesses that I may never have noticed otherwise and it has forced us to appreciate every breath. But 2001 tested me, and I really had to squint at times to see any good anywhere, in anything.

In the background MS kept creeping up on us. It kept slowly progressing, as always.

Our girls were growing up fast. Annie turned three, Aisling turned two and Sara was nearly one. My life was starting to get easy again. They were such fun and great friends and I loved being with them. They all slept through the night at this stage and I had more mental energy because I too could sleep once again. In November 2001, I started to seriously research MS and Parkinson's on the internet. I didn't know very much about them at all up to that point so I started reading and reading and reading. It became an obsession. I hated what I read, but I couldn't stop.

Initially, the learning curve was steep because I had to wade through much medical jargon, but I understood it. I was able to piece it all together somehow. The more I read and understood, the easier it was to read and understand more. I firmly concluded that MS stinks. Plain and simple. MS stinks. I didn't share my obsession with Noel. He knew that I was reading about it, but he wasn't interested in it. I concluded that he was smart because why know how awful MS can be when you might luck out and get it easy. The more I read, the more I realized that very few people with MS have an easy life. It was clear, MS stinks. It was equally clear that Parkinson's stinks and the chances of Neilus having it easy were also very slim.

Then came January 2002 and Noel started to slip fast.

Chapter 10

"Let perseverance be your engine and hope your fuel."
                                        H. Jackson Brown Jr.

At first, I only noticed his increased dependence on his cane around the house. It was no big deal initially, but I was aware that he was slipping a little. At the time, I was delighted that Mom's breast cancer was the best possible breast cancer there was. She told me that she didn't need a mastectomy, chemotherapy or radiation.

"Mary," she said, "It is only a little nothing."

My bubble didn't last long because I read about breast cancer and called her doctor. I discovered that she had a long road ahead of her, but I felt sure that she would get through it.

We spent many hours on the phone back then. When I was growing up she was always the ultimate optimist grounded in prayer. She was incredibly selfless and always the peacemaker. She was so glad that I didn't flip out. As long as I was okay, she promised that she would be fine. I was more than okay. I guided her through what to expect and all of the questions to ask her doctors. I told her how long things should take and how she would feel afterwards. I even told her that she would lose her hair, but then told her not to worry about it because it would grow back better.

Mom had the strangest view of her cancer. First, in her mind as always, was the firm belief that God never gives you more than you can handle because God is very good. Second, was sincere gratitude that she had cancer instead of anybody in her family. She figured that it was much easier to deal with it than to watch anybody she loved deal with it. In her mind, she was very lucky.

As is tradition in Ireland, her cancer was not discussed much and life went on as normal. I remember phoning home shortly before her mastectomy, when the family was gathered, and nobody seemed to have a care in the world. Mom liked that. I heard from friends of mine in nursing that she was the life and soul of the hospital, stunning people with cancer and those working with cancer, with her attitude.

After her mastectomy, she needed chemotherapy because her cancer had spread to her lymph nodes. She went the whole nine yards. They told her that she would probably feel tired and nauseous after each treatment. She told them that her daughter in the U.S. explained it all to her and then she went on to talk nonstop about her three granddaughters. Dad told her that chemotherapy could prove to be a useful diet. She laughed about that because she was always on the lookout for crazy diets.

Annie drove five hours, from Arranmore to Galway, to be with Mom for every treatment and as soon as she was done they would eat a three course meal and shop until the stores shut. Mom never felt nauseous and she didn't lose any weight. She did lose her hair and set a trend with head scarves.

After her chemotherapy, Mom was told that she had to go to Dublin for radiation therapy. I planned a trip home with my girls to surprise her on completion. As I was planning my trip back to Ireland, Noel was steadily declining in the background. It was spring 2002, and I remember watching him cut the grass. He was no longer able to do it without resting periodically because his legs kept giving in on him. It was time to confront the fact that Avonex was failing him.

I was not sure what to do at this point. Noel realized that he was slipping, but as always hc was completely fine about it. When I would ask him how he felt, he used to give me the biggest hug and tell me that he was perfectly fine. I said that I noticed that cutting the grass was getting difficult for him and he said that was just the way MS was. He said that he was mentally prepared for the worst and wanted to enjoy the fact that although he stumbled and had to rest a little, hc was still able to cut the grass. That was a great thing he claimed. I started to feel very uneasy about my upcoming trip home.

Noel and Mom always had a very special bond because they shared a similar view of life. Noel insisted that I went home for a month to be with Mom and promised that he would join us for the last two wccks. I hesitated. I asked him to go and see his neurologist before my flight just to set my mind at ease. He assured me that he was fine, but if that was what it would take for me to surprise my mom then he would go. Noel went to see his neurologist shortly before my flight home and was told that he was finc. My mind settled. I figured that I must just have been overreacting seeing as my mind was focused on Mom for so long. I felt totally relieved. Thank God everything was okay, I thought.

My three girls and I flew to Dublin in late April 2002. My girls were wonderful travelers. I suppose they were used to it. It is amazing me how accommodating people on an airplane can be when you travel with three kids under four. Everybody was more than happy to give us as much room as possible and move to a seat, far, far away. Traveling with my girls was better than traveling first class.

My youngest brother, Kevin, and his wife, Lisa, were living in Dublin, at the time, so we had a royal welcome. Annie was also there to greet us. As always it felt great to be in Ireland. We headed to Kevin and Lisa's house and planned to see Mom in the morning. Word had already slipped out that we had landed and were going to surprise her. I remember thinking that I could not wait until I would see her in the morning.

As soon as it was morning we went to St Luke's hospital in Dublin. It was a beautiful morning. Sunny and warm with a bright blue sky. I hate hospitals and this one reminded me of an old folk's home I worked for in Belfast during my year out from my studies. It had a particular scent that I hated. I desperately wanted to get Mom out of there.

My children had a ridiculous fear of elevators for the longest time and their phobia was at its peak at this time. Normally, I made them endure the elevator ride, insisting they must confront their fears in order to conquer them, but this was a special day, so we took the stairs. I needed to conserve all of my energy, and climbing a few flights of stairs with three young ones was considered a saving in my book. I saw Mom. She looked fresh-faced and was wearing a head scarf I sent her from the U.S.. We were incredibly happy so see each other. She was done! It was over!

Thank God for children. They stole our focus and had all sorts of stories for Grandma Maureen. Meanwhile, Granny Annie decided it was time to eat. We headed for the hospital cafeteria because Mom said that she had many people whom she felt she had to thank and say goodbye to. I felt strong and was so thankful that I could actually see her. I prayed that everything would be okay. I wasn't pretending to be strong anymore. I really was strong.

We started to have fun. The three girls were the life and soul of our fun. From Dublin, we headed to Galway and after a stint in Galway with Grandpa Vince, we headed to Arranmore. Grandpa Neilus had such a crazy welcome for all of us. He had every toy you could imagine for the girls, including a bouncy castle and a swing set. Luckily for me, Annie and Neilus never had a family of their own. I always told them that that was because I needed them more than anyone.

It was immediately obvious to me that Neilus' Parkinson's had progressed. His shake had become very apparent, but thank God he had the best possible Parkinson's. We all had fun together. It felt so good and we were looking forward to Noel joining us early in May.

Noel was finally due to arrive in a couple of days. He called me one night prior and told me that he was finding it difficult to walk. He assured me that it was no big deal. He explained that his biggest concern was preparing his parents to greet him at the airport in a wheelchair. He figured that he would definitely need a wheelchair for this visit because he was familiar with the walking distance required at the airport. He asked me if I could meet him with his parents to help make light of it all. We were used to wheelchairs from Disney and other parks in the U.S.. I asked him to describe his decline. He told me that he was getting better and starting to feel stronger because his neurologist gave him steroids. He didn't have to say any more. The fact that he went to his neurologist without me nagging him to death said it all. I told him not to worry about his parents. I assured him that I would organize a fanfare to greet him and with all of the commotion it was possible that his parents wouldn't even notice his wheelchair.

I hung up and could not wait to see him. This time, I even made light of the situation with Mom and Annie. I had toughened up a great deal in the last few years and was starting to reap the benefits.

Chapter 11

"Don't believe in miracles. Rely on them."

Anonymous

N oel is the only boy of four. He was always the pride and joy of his parents. They never accepted his MS very well by any means. It hit them very hard, especially his mother, Maura. She figured that he had suffered enough in life and for her, his MS was the last straw. She could not stand to think of him slowly deteriorating. She couldn't even pretend that she could. This put a great strain on their relationship because Noel hated to see his mother upset. He knew there was nothing he could do to fix it. Equally, it upset Maura that Noel could not relate to her pain. Noel, I suppose, is a typical man. His way of dealing with a problem is to provide a solution. His solution for his MS was acceptance and that was not easy for many. When he called his mom to say that he would need a wheelchair at the airport for the visit, I knew that it would deeply upset her. I also knew that no fanfare would hide his wheelchair from her because I understood that she was eagerly waiting to analyze his current condition.

I picked up the phone and called Maura and as expected, she was very upset. I told her that it wasn't easy, but it was important that we all remained calm and strong for Noel. He was genuinely handling the whole thing so well that I felt like it was the duty of everybody else to do the same for him. I knew that it was difficult for Maura and in many ways it was hardest on her most of all because she was not with him all of the time. If you are with somebody with MS all of the time you gradually adjust to their decline. It seemed that just being with Noel made it easier for me to accept. Distance however made it very difficult for Maura and distance also wreaked havoc on an imagination steeped in fear.

Maura and his dad wanted to meet Noel on their own in Dublin with no fanfare. I understood and respected their wishes so we agreed that the girls and I would head to Fahan and meet Noel at his parent's house after they picked him up. I am very fond of Noel's parents and am grateful that we have a very honest relationship. We always feel comfortable speaking our mind.

As soon as I saw Noel, it was instantly clear that he had slipped. He was now completely dependent on his cane and the distance that he could walk had greatly diminished. Also, his bladder was very weak. But Noel was high on life. He was so happy to see the girls and me and had many stories about traveling with a disability.

Noel's pet peeve in life is people's lack of consideration for others. Couple that with a disdain for incompetence and add a dash of impatience to understand why it was funny to hear how he had to wait on the plane for so

long after everybody else disembarked because somebody
forgot to get him a wheelchair. Noel learns fast. As soon
as we got back to the U.S. he bought his own chair. He
decided that he never wanted to wait for a wheelchair ever
again.

We had a lot of fun in Fahan. We knew that it was difficult for his parents, but everybody made the best of the
situation. After Fahan, we traveled to Galway and before
we knew it we were back in New Jersey.

Soon it was June 2002, and Noel continued to decline.
He could no longer cut the front lawn at all and to do the
back he needed to rest four or five times. It was very difficult to watch him, but the way he handled it was literally
beyond belief. He never ever complained. He was always
happy and fun to be with. I kept my vow to be strong for
him, but I confess I found it difficult at times.

As soon as Noel used to leave for work in the morning I
would gather the children and pray. It kept me sane. The
only time I felt truly at peace was when I prayed. The children loved it. I suppose children sense everything, especially ill-hidden tension. They liked it when I was calm.
That is what prayer did for me, it always calmed me. Obviously, I couldn't pray all day as I had much to tend to, but
my quiet moments were spent in prayer. Throughout all of
this I continued to meet the Moms Group on Wednesday
mornings at Nativity.

Many from the Moms Group were deeply concerned for
me at this point, but I was strong. I had a coping mechanism in place. Also, I had hope. I was starting to read about
people with MS on the internet who had taken their health
into their own hands. They described how they felt that the
medical community and MS societies had failed them.
Some were using bee stings, others were on a particular
diet and others were using histamine. There seemed to be a

whole array of options to explore.

It was very clear to me at this point that Avonex was not working for Noel. I read everything about Avonex and even Biogen advised people to come off it if they started to progress rapidly. I told Noel what I thought, but he told me more firmly than I would have liked, that he would not listen to my advice because I was not a neurologist. True, he had a very valid point. Noel really liked his neurologist at this stage and felt that he was getting the best possible treatment. He explained that he had a neurologist so that his neurologist could tell him what drugs to take and when to come off them. That was his neurologist's job, not mine, he insisted.

Noel honestly felt that it was futile to waste valuable time chasing a pipedream. He told me that people must go crazy trying to fight MS. He explained that it made much more sense to maximize every second he had with his family. He vowed that he would never make MS his life or undertake any quest to find a cure or indulge in any form of quackery. He insisted that he would let his neurologist decide what was best for him at every turn and he told me very firmly to leave it at that. Noel wanted to keep going at full speed for as long as possible without thinking about it. He asked me to accept his condition and to make the most of whatever we had and whatever was coming our way.

I loved Noel's strength, acceptance and world view. He held an unnerving conviction that he would pass the test of life regardless of circumstance and it was admirable. But, I could not let it be. Just as Noel had to live his way, I too, had to live mine. I told Noel that if I had MS, I would wear a histamine patch, eat everything raw and despite a ridiculous bee phobia I would sting myself daily, one hundred times if necessary. I told him that I would fight with everything I had. I wished that I had MS instead of him because I would fight hard and I would beat it. I was angry.

It is silly what people wish for. I mean, if I *was* granted a wish at that point in time, it would have been for me to have MS instead of Noel. How crazy a wish is that? Maybe it is an Irish trait to think that *somebody* has to have MS. To this day, Noel insists that he is delighted to have MS instead of me as if one of us absolutely had to have it. I wish that nobody in the world had MS, ever. I hate MS. And I also hate cancer. How could my mother ever have been grateful that she had cancer instead of anyone in her family? It doesn't make any sense to me. I would be grateful if nobody in the world had cancer, ever. That would be good. But, if I had MS, I told Noel again, at least I would fight it. I would fight like heck.

Noel laughed and told me that that was exactly why he was glad that I didn't have MS. It was better for us that it was he who had to deal with it instead of me. He told me that if I had MS I would turn it into an extremely unhealthy obsession.

"Let's enjoy every second of every day we have together. Let's not waste any of our time," he begged.

I was never quite sure if his coping mechanism for dealing with MS was a form of denial or a genuine gift of grace. As more time passed, I became convinced that Noel had the gift of grace. Having watched Noel over the years, I also became convinced that if there is a test of life, he has already passed it. And if he hasn't, God help the rest of us.

Every morning Noel would go to work and I would pray with the children to calm myself and in my spare time I used to read about MS on the internet. I could not let it be. I had to fight, so I read and I read and I read. I learned that MS is incredibly elusive. What works for one person may not work for somebody else. To further complicate the picture, I learned that it is difficult to definitively measure whether or not anything actually works for MS because it can always be argued that if the sufferer did absolutely nothing, their MS might have stopped progressing anyway, out of the blue, for no reason. MS is tricky. It stops and starts, often without reason. For me to confront Noel again I needed something that was definitely working for everyone with MS, across the board. I needed a miracle.

I kept telling the Moms Group that there had to be somebody somewhere who knew how to treat MS effectively. They used to nod sympathetically at me. I am certain they thought that I was losing my mind, but I knew that I wasn't. I was just searching. Then, one morning I found what I was looking for.

I often look back on that morning in early August 2002. I was tired and had shut myself off from the Moms Group to make time for my search. I started to skip our Wednesday morning sessions. Many from the group phoned me daily, even when I didn't return calls. They persisted and often called round to surprise me. They were always more than welcome. I was simply preoccupied, at the time, because there was so much to read.

One particular morning, Noel went to work and I prayed. His balance was absolutely dreadful. He could hardly get off the couch without three or four heaves and when he finally managed to stand, he often fell over. I had plans to buy him a walker for the house and was seriously considering moving our bedroom to the ground floor because it was a nightmare watching him climb the stairs at night. It was a scary time. However, as always, Noel's spirits were great and he was quite prepared for a permanent wheelchair.

"A wheelchair is not a big deal," he said.

I laugh about this now because it is a little bit funny. It used to take me so long to calm myself before leaving the house for various classes or appointments for the kids that I often misplaced things, especially my keys. I used to lose my keys three to four times a day. Like many people from Ireland, I was trained at a young age to pray to St. Anthony if ever I lost anything because he is the saint in charge of lost and found. Amazingly, it often worked for me. Over-tired and leaving the house with the three children I used to automatically ask St. Anthony to help me find my keys and I would find them. This particular morning on finding my keys I laughed and said to the children that it would be great if St. Anthony would invest his time more wisely and find what I really needed. I really needed to find the right treatment for Noel because I knew that Avonex was completely failing him, even harming him. So, I asked St. Anthony to find the right treatment for Noel.

I was living moment to moment, but that one stands out. If by any possible chance I had St. Anthony's ear, talk about wasting my moment. It is like the wasted wish, wishing that I had MS instead of Noel. I must train myself to think bigger and more positively. I should have asked St. Anthony to find a cure for MS and put an end to all of the craziness. To tell the truth, I don't know if St. Anthony ever heard me, but I like to imagine that he did. It would be a great story if he really did. I have since asked him to stop messing around and find a cure and although he hasn't found one yet, I will keep asking.

I do know for certain that I was thinking about buying a walker for Noel, at the time, and I was trying to remember for days where I bought his cane because I liked the service they provided. I had basically given up on remembering and had intended to shop elsewhere that afternoon. Before I left the house, after my prayer to St. Anthony, I logged out of the internet to free up my phone line, and noticed a popup window with the address and phone number of

Town and Country Pharmacy in Ridgewood. That was the name and number I was trying to remember and find for days because that was where I bought his cane. I dialed the number immediately to inquire about various walking aids for Noel and the owner, John Herr, answered the phone.

When we bought Noel's cane in Town and Country, they were very helpful. They went that extra mile for us. It is not nice to have to buy a cane, but they made it seem okay. I recognized John's voice when he answered the phone. I began by explaining that my husband had MS and John interrupted me. I wanted to thank him for the wonderful service he provided when I bought the cane and ask him about walkers and all different types of walking aids. I knew that he would be able to tell me a great deal about them and I also knew that if he didn't stock exactly what I needed that he would know a man who did. I never had any of that conversation with him. The first thing he asked me on hearing that my husband had MS was whether or not my husband was taking LDN. I said no and asked him what LDN was.

He told me about a customer and friend of his, Fritz Bell, who hosted a website at www.goodshape.net. Fritz was married to Polly and Polly had very severe MS. Her MS was progressing rapidly, but it completely stopped progressing since she started taking LDN two years previously. John told me that he compounded LDN for Polly and although he confessed that he didn't know a great deal about the drug, he did know that it was a safe bet because it was cheap and had no known side-effects. He said that he thought LDN would be worth a shot for Noel. He told me that Mr. Bell (also known as Mr. Goodshape) had a lot more information on his website. John also explained that Noel might have difficulty getting a prescription for the drug because it was not medically recognized as a treatment for

MS. He said that some people who could not persuade their neurologists, asked their primary care physician (regular doctor) to prescribe the drug for them off-label because it was already FDA approved at a much higher dose for heroin addicts. Before I hung up, John finished by telling me that if I needed any help in convincing Noel's neurologist to prescribe LDN, he was more than willing to help me in any way possible. I deeply appreciated his concern and willingness to help. Once again he went the extra mile for a stranger. I decided to investigate and could not believe what I read.

Even for an optimist, it sounded too good to be true.

Chapter 12

*"Do all the good you can, by all the means you can, in all
the ways you can, in all the places you can, at all the times
you can, to all the people you can, as long as you can."*
Anonymous

I logged on to the internet and went to Goodshape's site.
There was a lot of information on the benefits of histamine, but I had already presented histamine as an option
to Noel and knew that he wasn't interested. I was specifically looking for information on LDN and then I found it.
Goodshape's site had a link to the official LDN website.
This is the first thing I read. I could not take it in initially:

"Clinically the results are strongly suggestive of efficacy. Ninety-eight to 99% of people treated with LDN experience no more disease progression, whether the disease
category is relapsing-remitting or chronic progressive. Dr.
Bihari has more than seventy people with MS in his practice

and all are stable over an average of three years. The original patient on LDN for MS, now on it for seventeen years, has not had an attack or disease progression for twelve years since the one missed month that led to an attack.

In addition, 2,000 or more people with MS have been prescribed LDN by their family MDs or their neurologists based on what they have read on the LDN website or heard about in internet chat rooms focused on MS. Many such patients with MS, not under Dr. Bihari's care, use the e-mail link on the LDN website to ask questions. Many prescribing physicians do not generally know about LDN.

Only once has a patient reported disease progression while on LDN. In this case, it showed itself five days after he had started the drug. The onset of the episode had apparently preceded the start of LDN.

In addition to the apparent ability of LDN to stop disease progression, approximately two-thirds of MS patients starting LDN have some symptomatic improvement generally apparent within the first few days. There are two types of such improvement.

One is reduction in spasticity when this is present, sometimes allowing easier ambulation when spasticity in the legs has been a prominent element of a patient's difficulty in walking or standing. This is unlikely to represent a direct effect of LDN on the disease process, but rather reduction in the irritability in nervous tissue surrounding plaques. Endorphins have been shown to reduce irritability of nervous tissue, e.g., by reducing seizures in patients with epilepsy.

The other area of symptomatic improvement in some patients is a reduction in MS-related fatigue. This is, also, not likely due to a direct effect on the MS disease process, but rather an indirect one caused by restoration of normal endorphin levels improving energy.

Patients who are in the midst of an acute exacerbation when they start LDN have generally shown rapid resolution of the attack. In two patients, chronic visual impairment due to old episodes of optic neuritis has shown fluctuating improvement.

It should be emphasized that in spite of the plentitude of clinical experience described above, in the absence of a formal clinical trial of LDN in MS, these results cannot be considered scientific, but rather anecdotal. A clinical trial, preferably by a pharmaceutical company with some experience with MS, is clearly needed to determine whether these results can be replicated. If they can be, they are likely to lead to widespread use of this extremely non-toxic drug in the treatment of MS."

That was my starting point. At that time, I was well aware of the chances of the standard MS drugs slowing the progression of Relapsing Remitting MS only, and none of them came remotely close. This was saying that LDN does not slow the progression; it actually stops the progression 98-99% of the time, regardless of the type of MS. It was unbelievable. I instantly decided that I didn't want to know anything more about LDN until I thoroughly investigated the doctor behind these claims, Dr. Bernard Bihari. I also wanted to quickly figure out who was profiting from the website advertising these bold claims.

I performed an internet wide search on Dr. Bernard Bihari which led me to the home page of the LDN webpage that was linked to Goodshape's site. I laughed because it took me a while to travel that circle. I noticed that Dr. Bihari's Curriculum Vitae (CV) was part of the site. I thought that it read very well. It said that he achieved his MD from Harvard and listed his New York State Medical License Number 088158. I used that number to verify part of his CV with the New York State Education Department. I found his record and it read:

Name : BIHARI BERNARD
Address : NEW YORK NY
Profession : MEDICINE
License No: 088158
Date of Licensure : 09/07/62
Additional Qualification : A - Certified to practice
acupuncture
Status : REGISTERED
Registered through last day of : 10/09
Medical School: HARVARD UNIVERSITY Degree
Date : 06/13/1957

I continued to investigate and read on his CV that he was board-certified since 1970. I confirmed that information with the American Board of Psychiatry and neurology. His CV also stated that he was an attending physician at Beth Israel Medical Center in New York, so I phoned Beth Medical and confirmed that information. I concluded that it was difficult to believe that Dr. Bihari was a quack because his credentials were solid.

Then I checked out the website itself to see who was sponsoring it. I was again impressed to learn that it was a nonprofit website:

"This website is sponsored by Advocates for Therapeutic Immunology. The purpose of this website is to provide information to patients and physicians about important therapeutic breakthroughs in advanced medical immunology. The authors of this site do not profit from the sale of LDN or from website traffic, and are in no way associated with any pharmaceutical manufacturer or pharmacy."

I became convinced that Dr. Bihari was not a quack and was not trying to make a fast dollar. I was intrigued, to say the least, so I decided to find out what LDN actually was.

I learned that LDN stood for Low Dose Naltrexone. Naltrexone Hydrochloride is a white powder chemical compound. It is a drug that is listed in the Physician's Desk Reference (PDR) and is an approved treatment for substance abuse, such as heroin addiction. Since it is listed in the PDR, doctors may use their own judgment in deciding whether to prescribe Naltrexone off-label to other individuals, such as those with MS.

Naltrexone is marketed in generic form, Naltrexone Hydrochloride, under the trade names Revia, Nodict, Vivtrol and Depade. Although it is primarily a narcotic antagonist, it has also been shown to reduce craving and consumption for some patients who are alcohol dependent. The FDA approved standard dose given to patients with a substance abuse problem is 50 mg Naltrexone.

At first I didn't understand how a drug used for substance abuse could help people with MS. Then I learned that Naltrexone in different doses, does completely different things. At a low dose of 4.5 mg, Dr. Bihari was using LDN to boost the immune systems of his patients. Such thinking flies in the face of conventional MS thinking because the standard MS medications work on suppressing the immune system based on the theory that people with MS have an overactive immune system. Dr. Bihari was challenging all conventional views of MS by trying to boost the immune system as opposed to suppressing it. I liked that because I had seen conventional medicine fail Noel.

So, how does LDN actually work? Imagine you are a heroin addict. You want to get over your addiction so you take the FDA approved 50 mg Naltrexone daily. Some addicts actually take up to 200 mg daily. Then you have a weak moment and decide to take a hit of heroin. Despite the hit, you won't get high, because at 50 mg, Naltrexone will block the opioid receptors in your brain for twenty-four hours. It is hoped that one would stop taking the heroin thanks to Naltrexone preventing the expected high.

At a low dose of 4.5 mg, Naltrexone blocks the same opioid receptors, but only for three or four hours. During that time, the pituitary and adrenal glands respond to the inability of those receptors and flood the body with three times more endorphins than usual. Although the short blockade ends, the increased endorphins last most of the day and boost the immune system enough to ensure it stops attacking one's own tissues. That is why it works for such a wide range of autoimmune diseases.

Now imagine you are a drug addict with MS. If you take the FDA approved 50 mg Naltrexone for your addiction, your MS will get worse because you are blocking endorphin reception for too long. At a high dose, Naltrexone will not rectify a disturbed immune system. So, if you have a drug problem plus an autoimmune disease or cancer even, it would be wise to avoid taking Naltrexone at 50 mg. There is no point curing an addiction for a clean cancer death. That piece of important information was not picked up in the FDA trial that approved Naltrexone for various addictions. And once a drug has been FDA approved, it is very difficult to get funding for further testing.

I was curious what prompted Dr. Bihari's thinking so I read more and dug deeper. I learned that Dr. Bihari's early work consisted of helping those afflicted with drug and alcohol abuse in New York City. From there, in the 1980's, his work extended to the HIV and AIDS community. It is during this time, after years of experimenting with Naltrexone dosing, he discovered the therapeutic effects of LDN for HIV and AIDS. He observed that addicts with HIV did not develop full blown AIDS when they took a low dose of Naltrexone. From what I know of the man, I believe that his heart lay in helping the AIDS epidemic and that he stumbled into helping the MS community serendipitously.

In 1988, his daughter's best friend, Chris Lombardi, was diagnosed with MS and because Dr. Bihari had seen the capability of LDN to boost the immune system in his HIV and AIDS patients, he prescribed LDN for Chris. He believed that HIV and AIDS and MS had one thing in common. They were diseases based on disturbed immune systems. It was more than plausible, in Dr. Bihari's mind, that LDN would work for MS seeing as it was showing great promise in HIV and AIDS patients in his practice.

Chris was twenty-two in 1988 and there was no treatment whatsoever for MS. Dr. Bihari prescribed 3 mg LDN and she took it for five years with no progression. Then, she went out of state and her LDN supply ran out. She felt so good she figured that she didn't need LDN anymore so she stopped taking it. Within a month or so, her MS started to flare up again so she immediately resumed LDN treatment. Chris was the first MS patient on LDN and a remarkable testimony to its benefits.

For many years since 1988, Dr. Bihari dedicated himself to the AIDS crisis, but through word of mouth the potential that LDN had for MS spread, and he was contacted by more and more people suffering with MS. At first the word spread very slowly. By the time I actually followed his story through and picked up the phone to speak with him he had less than eighty patients with MS, but they were all stable regardless of the type of MS they were diagnosed with.

I remember picking up the nerve to call Dr. Bihari. His address and phone number were part of his CV that was posted on the LDN site. Noel was at work and my three girls were napping. I had no idea what to expect, but I was more than pleasantly surprised.

Chapter 13

*"People may forget what you said, but they will
never forget how you made them feel."*
                    Carl W. Buechner

My first surprise was that Dr. Bihari actually answered the phone himself. I introduced myself and explained that I had been reading about his work on the internet and wanted to talk to him about it before presenting it all to Noel. Dr. Bihari was very friendly. I was honest with him and told him that it sounded too good to be true. I explained that I didn't want to play on Noel's emotions and I couldn't trust my own. I had to be very certain of my information before I even thought about raising Noel's hopes. Dr. Bihari completely understood and proceeded to assure me that all I read was true. He started at the very beginning and explained everything to me in terms that I could understand. His manner was laid back and relaxed. He was easy to talk with and listen to and I felt his compassion. He told me about his work with the AIDS and HIV community, but I wasn't interested in any of that at the time. I just wanted to know about LDN and MS.

Dr. Bihari told me that he believed everybody with an autoimmune disorder has low levels of endorphins. Before he explained what endorphins were, he told me what exactly an autoimmune disease is. He said that the word "auto" is the Greek word for self. The immune system is a complicated network that normally works to defend the body and eliminate infections, but if a person has an autoimmune disease, the immune system mistakenly attacks itself, targeting the cells, tissues, and organs of a person's own body. There are many different autoimmune diseases, and they can each affect the body in different ways. For example, the autoimmune reaction is directed against the brain and spinal cord in Multiple Sclerosis, and against the gut in Crohn's disease.

I had read on the internet that there are many theories as to what MS actually is and it is even debated as to whether or not it is autoimmune. Also, the definitions and naming of various types and stages of MS is highly debated. Everything about MS is debated. It is incredibly elusive. That is what makes it even more frustrating, but Dr. Bihari firmly believed that MS is an autoimmune disease. He believed that is why LDN stops it in its tracks.

Dr. Bihari continued and explained that just as the sex hormone, testosterone, controls sexual function, endorphins control and regulate the immune system. Dr. Bihari said that endorphins are produced nightly. He believed that endorphin production had a biological clock which people call a circadian rhythm, and that that internal human biological clock dictates that most of our endorphins are produced nightly. He calculated that the best time to take LDN would be between 9:00 p.m. and 2:00 a.m.. He said that LDN, if taken nightly, causes endorphin production to triple, bringing the levels up to normal, and once normal, the immune system stops attacking itself. Dr. Bihari claimed that if endorphin production was regulated, the endorphins would be able to control and regulate the immune system. Hence, the immune system would no longer attack one's self. He told me that was why none of his MS patients had progressed. It was that simple.

"LDN is not a cure for MS," he insisted. He stated that LDN would only remove the last three months of damage, if Noel was lucky, but it seemed to be universal in stopping MS disease progression.

Many years have passed since that phone call. Today, most people on LDN, especially with MS, follow the Dr. Bihari protocol religiously and take their LDN between 9:00 p.m. and 2:00 a.m.. Most of the anecdotal evidence surrounding the success of LDN with MS came from people who take LDN at night. Therefore, if I had MS, I would follow the protocol that best proved (albeit anecdotally) effectiveness.

However, since my conversation with Dr. Bihari, it has been highly debated as to whether or not endorphin production has a circadian rhythm. Beta-endorphin levels are definitely highest from 6 – 10:00 a.m. according to Naber et al. Also, Farsang et al. and Petraglia et al. agree that the levels are highest in the morning and lowest in the evening. And, Dent et al. published that beta endorphin levels are lowest between 10:00 p.m. and 3:30 a.m., and highest from 4:00 a.m. to 10:00 a.m.. So, it is agreed that most of our endorphins are produced sometime before dawn. It is also agreed that most people will not set their alarm for 4:00 a.m. (which would seem to be the perfect time) to take LDN. Therefore, I have to conclude that the best time to take LDN has to be before bed. Is that the only time to take it?

No. I know people who have felt much benefit by taking LDN at different times of the day. To take that risk however, would have to depend on the fight being fought.

The whole debate surrounding the best time to take LDN emerged because a small minority of people who took LDN at night found it difficult to sleep. Typically, most people adjusted after a week or so of sleepless nights, but sometimes the problem persisted. I have heard a couple of wonderful stories from wonderful people who take their LDN in the morning and still manage to reap many benefits. Would they reap more if they took it at night? I have to say that I think so, but yet, a morning dose does seem to increase endorphin production enough for some people. If I had MS, I would try LDN at night first because that is what has worked for the majority of people thus far and it has been proven that endorphin levels peak before dawn and I would want my body to produce as much endorphins as possible. If I experienced sleep disturbance, I would realize that many people have and that it generally passes. I actually love to hear stories of initial sleep disturbance and vivid dreams when somebody starts LDN because, in my mind, that means that LDN is doing its thing. However, if the problem persisted for over a month, I would try LDN in the morning or at a different time of day. I would prefer do that than abandon ship. And who knows, a large scale trial one day might prove that timing doesn't matter in the slightest. For now, however, based on the evidence at hand, I would play it safe.

My phone conversation with Dr. Bihari continued. I proceeded to tell him about my uncle Neilus and his Parkinson's. To my amazement, Dr. Bihari told me that although Parkinson's was medically documented with unknown etiology, he believed that Parkinson's might be an autoimmune disease. He told me that because of his success with HIV, AIDS and MS he started branching out into a whole spectrum of what he considered to be autoimmune diseases. He explained that he was very thankful for others' use of the internet because it made it possible for him to reach so many more people than ever before. He told me that he had three Parkinson's patients on LDN for over a year and that although it was too early for him to say for sure that it worked, he assured me that it looked very promising. LDN was worth a try for Parkinson's, he said, based on the fact that there are no serious side-effects and it is a very inexpensive therapy.

Our conversation continued to naturally flow. It was a long phone call. I think that I spoke with Dr. Bihari for over forty-five minutes in total. I asked him about breast cancer and I explained to him that my mom had a recent mastectomy and had just finished her chemotherapy and radiation therapy. Again he was most eager to share. He told me that he was actually taking LDN himself since 1992 to prevent cancer because it was prevalent in his family. He told me that he had twenty women with breast cancer on LDN for five years and all were still in remission. He said that typically half of them would have had a reoccurrence by now without LDN.

It was difficult to believe what I was hearing, but I knew by talking with him that he believed what he was saying and it seemed that he had great reason to do so.

I thanked him at the end of our call and asked him if I should pay him. He refused payment. He said that he was delighted I had found the website on LDN and that he was positive LDN would greatly help my family. He explained that any doctor could prescribe LDN off-label for his or her patients and told me he was happy to share his information with me and wished me well. He added that if Noel's neurologist or doctor wanted to speak with him, he would gladly share his case studies with them. Before I hung up, he asked, that should my family decide to take LDN that I would make sure it was compounded as described on the LDN website. He assured me that it was an easy thing to do and that any compounding pharmacy could do it if instructed properly, but it was important that it was compounded correctly for it to work.

I hung up and sat quiet for a little while. I decided not to say anything to anyone just yet because I needed time for everything to sink in. I also needed to read more.

I believed Dr. Bihari at this point, but I wanted to hear what others were saying. I was well aware of my ability to be overly optimistic and I wanted to keep myself in check. I had to be absolutely positive of everything before speaking with Noel, Neilus and Mom.

I called my brother that evening. He was an established doctor at this stage, so I asked him if LDN could possibly do Noel any harm. To my amazement, Phil was most interested in my findings. Phil specializes in NaProTECH-NOLOGY, a new reproductive and gynecologic science which has been developed at the Pope Paul VI Institute for the Study of Human Reproduction. The Institute has created a standardized modification of the Billings Ovulation Method and called it the Creighton Model FertilityCare System. Phil told me that they were already using LDN at much higher doses to boost fertility for some couples. At the time, Phil had no doubt that LDN somehow boosts fertility by boosting endorphins, and he assured me that at 4.5 mg it would do Noel no harm. Phil told me that LDN for MS was consistent with a fundamental guiding principle of medicine. "Primum non nocere" or "First do no harm." Phil believed I had nothing to lose and that maybe I was on the right track, so I continued to investigate.

It is interesting to note that since my first conversation

with Phil about LDN in August 2002, he gradually incorpo-
rated Dr. Bihari's 4.5 mg LDN protocol into his fertility
practice with astounding results. The lower dose of
Naltrexone worked better than the higher doses he had previously used for other patients. To date, some women who
used LDN to help them conceive, actually stayed on LDN
for the entire duration of their pregnancy with no side-
effects but one: A healthy baby. LDN has helped many
women with fertility problems. Today it seems like common sense to link fertility issues with a disturbed immune
system, but that was not always the case.

Before I continue, I would like to place Dr. Ian Zagon
in this puzzle. There has been, at times, heated debate on
the internet as to who actually discovered the therapeutic
effects of LDN. Some people insist it was Dr. Bihari and
others insist it was Dr. Zagon. Both men are heroes and to
compare them makes no sense. Ian S. Zagon, Ph D., is Pro-
fessor in neuroscience and Anatomy in Penn State College
of Medicine in Pennsylvania. He has been doing laboratory
research and pursuing all of the ins and outs surrounding
opioid blockade and endorphin function in mammals
(mainly rodents) in great detail for over twenty years. It is
entirely possible that Dr. Zagon and his colleagues' research was, in fact, the inspiration for Dr. Bihari's vision to
apply Low Dose Naltrexone to humans.

In 1984, Dr. Zagon and Patricia McLoughlin filed for
U.S. patent number 4,689,332 on the use of opioid antago-
nists such as Naltrexone, as growth regulators. Controlling
cancer growth using Low Dose Naltrexone was a major
part of their research. As part of this process, Dr. Zagon
provided the patent office with dosages of Naltrexone that
humans could use.

Using a weight basis of rats and mice, Dr. Zagon proposed that 3-10 mg/day of Naltrexone would yield a cancer

growth retardation, and a dosage of 20 -30 or higher mg/day would block opioid receptors all day and enhance growth.

They sent in their first paper on this to SCIENCE on March 21, 1983 and it was published August 12, 1983 (SCIENCE 221:671-673,1983). It was all about cancer. Their next paper was sent in on May 23, 1983 to SCIENCE and published September 16, 1983 (SCIENCE 221:1179-1180, 1983). These were historic papers because they provided evidence that the endogenous opioids i.e. endorphins, (not exogenous opioids like heroin) were cancer growth regulators. Naltrexone was proven to have the ability to enhance the body's own machinery to stimulate or repress cancer appearance/growth or body/organ growth, in mice.

It was around this time that Dr. Bihari started to use the off-label option to leap forward clinically rather than having to follow the gradual steps of careful research and punctilious scientific proof. Dr. Bihari's actions were legal and open to every physician and in this case much more has been gained than lost. For years, Dr. Bihari tried to get funding for a proper scientific trial, but in the meantime he legally prescribed the drug off-label for patients whom he knew did not have enough time to wait and were all out of options anyway. All of this led to Dr. Bihari's initial human clinical trial of LDN in HIV/AIDS in 1985-86 and subsequent application for U.S. patent number 4,888,346 on LDN to treat AIDS, in December 1987. Dr. Bihari deserves credit not only for LDN's utilization in HIV/AIDS, but also for LDN's clinical applications across a spectrum of categories including autoimmune diseases and human cancers. Dr. Bihari currently owns six patents on LDN use, including patent number 6,586,443 which he filed in 1994 and was granted in 2003, on LDN to treat MS. I am truly grateful that the efforts and passion of Dr. Zagon et al., in the laboratory, probably fuelled Dr. Bihari's passion to script LDN for his patients. Everybody is a hero in this story. When I thank Dr. Bihari for bringing LDN to the people, I am by no means discrediting the work of Dr. Zagon et al..

Back then in 2002, I was still not convinced of the merits of LDN. The only internet message board that discussed LDN at the time was Goodshape's, so I decided to thoroughly investigate his site.

Chapter 14

"Nothing in life is to be feared.
It is only to be understood."

Marie Curie

A message board is a meeting place on the internet where people with a common interest can share their views and experience. To be honest, at the time, I thought that such boards were only for people who couldn't relate in the real world. I thought that internet "chat rooms" were only for people who needed to hide behind a computer screen. But I was intrigued by the Goodshape site because John, the pharmacist from Town and Country in Ridgewood knew him. I lurked for a while and read what people had to say. I had friends whom I could have talked to if I needed to, but the internet provided something different. It provided an instant community of people in a similar position to mine, all fighting the same enemy.

When I first started posting on Goodshape's site I felt like "Mary no friends" because it was clear that my friends and family could not understand the issues that these people behind the screen could. I actually started to enjoy conversing with Goodshape and members of his site. I looked forward to getting home in the evenings to hear what was new or who had responded to my latest query. It was addictive. I heard many stories about LDN. They were all positive and I admired Goodshape for hosting the group. I even related to his circumstance as he, too, was fighting for his spouse whom he loved more than anything in the whole world. Polly was on LDN for two years at this time and she had not progressed despite her chronic diagnosis.

Goodshape wrote that he was also taking LDN as a cancer preventative and many people from the board shared heart wrenching stories that could only have been true.

Things were really happening on the Goodshape board. People with MS had hope and they inspired me so I told them my story. I told them that I was happily married to a headstrong man who had a solid conviction that he would carry his cross his way, with pride, and whose latest at the time was to explain to me that the best anyone in life can hope for is the ability to play out their hand with dignity. I shared with them that I had three children under four and that I was convinced of the merits of LDN, but knew that I would have a difficult job convincing Noel to even think about it. I asked for help and I was inundated with positive support and creative ideas. I could not believe the accuracy with which these strangers understood my predicament and I was astounded at their eagerness to help a complete stranger. I have to say, I was very moved.

They forewarned me of potential nightmare dealings

with neurologists and doctors but assured me that the fight was worth it in the end. LDN is the best possible treatment for MS was always the bottom line and they insisted that I never gave up.

I dug some more because I could not help but think that if LDN was so great, then why on earth was it such a secret? I questioned why Noel's neurologist didn't know about this. After all, he attended most of the MS meetings in New York along with the best MS experts in the world. It seemed logical to assume that if there was anything worth knowing about LDN then he would know about it. I deduced that if Noel's neurologist knew about LDN then Noel would have been on it, so I figured that Noel's neurologist was not aware of LDN and if he was aware of it, then it was obvious that he was not convinced of its merits. I also questioned why in the world nothing was published about LDN and MS at the time, but I don't understand the mechanics of publishing in the medical world. I can only assume that it is not very easy for a cheap, generic drug, with no side-effects and outrageous promise to get published. It was evident that I had more loose ends to tie up before sharing with family and friends because I knew that I had to be prepared to answer the obvious questions.

I posted my concerns on Goodshape's site and the plot started to thicken and my blood started to boil. Initially, I refused to believe that the world was so corrupt. I refused to believe what I read and part of me still does. A big part of me still cannot buy into this theory that is now believed by many to be true.

It was strongly suggested that the reason LDN had not hit the masses was because the drug companies dishing out the expensive drugs to MS patients stood to lose far too much money. It was spelled out to me that they make a nice profit tending to MS victims and that they were acting on their interests behind the scenes. It was strongly implied that the MS drug companies were actively preventing LDN from hitting the masses. Granted MS therapies are expensive and hence lucrative. Avonex is about $1200 a month compared to $35 a month for LDN, but I still didn't buy into this theory because I felt that it was based on paranoia. Maybe at first I did because I wanted somebody to blame, but as soon as I thought about it in depth I rejected it.

I immediately understood why Dr. Bihari had problems getting the drug into a scientific trial in the U.S.. It made business sense to me. LDN is a cheap generic drug. It is already FDA approved at ten times the dose, so it holds no monetary incentive for any pharmaceutical or U.S. Government body to run a series of expensive trials because it is generic, which means that anybody can sell it when they prove how good it is. Actually, the U.S. Government would save millions in the long run if even one tenth of what Dr. Bihari claims to be true was in fact true, because more people would be able to work and require less from the state. Corporate America however has a short term view of profit and works against the potential of a cheap drug despite the hope it holds for its citizens. That is a sad and tragic reality. But, were the big bad profit crazy drug companies actually actively stopping LDN getting out there? I didn't and I still don't believe that.

The problem I have with that theory is that the LDN community is too small. We are not big or scary enough yet to make any drug company take us seriously.

As far as I could see, in 2002, there were a handful of LDN advocates who saw LDN work. MS however is very elusive, so the same number of people could just as easily have been saying that the best way to stop MS progress is to pat your head and rub your tummy three times daily. The enigmatic world of MS provides a fertile breeding ground for quackery.

With regard to reaching the masses with LDN though, I firmly believe that there is no bad guy actively trying to prevent it from happening. I can see how the good guys, such as the MS societies, whose duty it is to help people with MS could be perceived as the bad guys simply because they openly want as little as possible to do with LDN. However, I believe that the real problem with getting anybody to seriously investigate the potential of LDN, particularly in the U.S., comes down to two major things. It lacks financial incentive and equally it lacks credibility. It is too simple a theory, too ridiculous to believe. I mean, even to me, an optimist by nature, with my back against the wall it was unbelievable. Despite credibility, the laws governing an out of patent, generic drug need to be changed so that they provide financial incentive for pharmaceutical companies to consider investing in clinical trials to prove a new use for an old drug.

When I look at the situation in Ireland, I see that the Government pays for all of the expensive MS medications for each person who decides to take them. In Ireland 6000 people have MS and about 2000 of them use a standard MS therapy. Anybody can do the math, 1200 Euro a month per person versus 30 Euro a month. Of course the Irish Government would prefer to pay for the LDN monthly and have less people dependent on them. They have been presented with a proposal to do a trial on LDN for MS and stand to save millions yearly. The only reason they did not set up a trial on receipt of the proposal has to be credibility (although a skeptic would question whether or not the Government is in bed with the pharmaceutical companies).

An LDN trial requires a leap of faith because the Governments don't want to risk funding an actual trial despite the potential it holds for future savings, not to mention future lives.

Getting back to August 2002, I had reached a point where I felt that I had thoroughly investigated LDN and I decided that it was time to present the information to Noel.

Chapter 15

"A man can be happy with any woman
as long as he does not love her."

Oscar Wilde

The best definition of love I ever heard came from Chris Rock, an American comedian. He said that unless you have thought about murder then you have never been in love.

In August 2002, Noel and I fell deeply in love. ADP was still reeling from the effects of the terrorist attack on the Twin Towers on September 11th 2001. Every month there were more and more cut backs so Noel's job was not secure and the prospect of us having to move back to Ireland became very real. Neither of us wanted to move because New Jersey had become our home. We loved all that it had to offer, especially for our children. We love the way of life and the positive openness of the people. Also, we have a wonderful network of friends with whom we have a lot of fun.

In the midst of all the work stress, the onslaught of Noel's MS continued. It was relentless. Also, the steroids started to lose their magic. Noel developed a level of immunity to steroids. Since then, I have learned that this is quite common.

One evening, Noel said that his worst symptom was his weak bladder. His balance was dreadful and I remember I could hear his left leg drag on the carpet when he walked around the house with his cane. He also fell quite often and had great difficulty getting up again. When he slept, his legs twitched every couple of minutes and I remember too, that he used to exercise his hands more. It was apparent that his hands were starting to become affected.

But, as the month passed, things got worse. MS stole our ability to be intimate. That put a great strain on our relationship because there are often times we rely on intimacy to communicate. There are no words for some situations. Overall, things were very tense.

One day in late August, Noel came home from work. He grabbed a beer and as always he spent the first half an hour rolling around the floor playing with the children. I told him that we needed to talk.

I think that everyone hates hearing those words, especially after a hostile day at work, so Noel ignored me. So, I just started to talk. I told him all about LDN as he wrestled with the children. He said nothing, so I told him it all again. He still said nothing and once again I repeated my thoughts. He finally looked at me and asked me where I found all of my information. He was visibly annoyed at my persistence. I told him about all of my virtual friends in cyberspace and could tell that he thought I had lost my mind. I expected that. I proceeded to tell him about Dr. Bihari and the phone call I had with him. Noel said that if there was any truth in what I was saying then his neurologist would know about LDN. I explained that it was quite possible that his neurologist did not know about it. I told him that LDN was relatively new for MS and not clinically proven, but it was cheap with no side-effects, so in my book we had nothing to lose by trying it.

In Noel's mind he had everything to lose he said because it would be the start of a million different goose chases I would send him on in search of a non-existent cure. He decided he had to nip all of the nonsense in the bud and enjoy whatever time he had, doing whatever he could do. He told me that he understood it was difficult for me, but added that I really had to accept his MS and face the fact that things were only going to get a whole lot worse. I was livid. Then he got mad. I really wanted to kill him. Without question, Chris Rock would have considered us very much in love.

I explained to Noel that just as he wanted me to accept his decline with grace, I wanted him to fight back with everything he had. We were head to head and neither of us was willing to give in. It was too important from both perspectives to budge on this one. It was a very tough situation.

During this time a very good friend of mine from the Moms group, Rachel Jones, was preparing to move to Ohio. Her husband was having difficulty finding work in New Jersey and wanted to move back to his roots. Rachel didn't want to move and was very stressed out at the time. Actually, despite the impact September 11th had on many of the Moms Group and our families, as a group we became tighter than ever.

I called over to Tia the morning after I told Noel about LDN, and Rachel was there. Most of the Moms Group turned to Tia in a crisis. She was warm and non judgmental.

That made her an easy person to confide in. I used to tease her that she was just crazy enough to make me feel sane. She told me that she liked to embrace her craziness and didn't like the fact that hanging out with me made her feel like she belonged in the sane category. The three of us, Tia, Rachel and I, were very close, so I told them the whole story. They knew something was going on with me for a while, but I will never forget their faces. They didn't know what to make of the LDN story. I will always love them because they helped me despite being convinced I was crazy. Even though they thought I had lost my mind, they took my children and told me to go and do whatever I had to do. They told me to follow through with my instincts and not to worry about the children. I left my little ones with them and went home to log on to the internet to e-mail a letter to Noel.

I told him that I loved him. I explained that I was worn out and could not stand fighting with him any longer. It was exhausting. I told him that the decision to try LDN had to be his decision because he was the one with MS. I pointed out that I didn't want to stress him out any more. I wrote that if he didn't want to take LDN, then he didn't have to. I told him that I was done arguing and asked him what he wanted for dinner.

That is something that MS taught me. It is now very important to me not to waste time fighting or arguing. I used to be able to hold a grudge for a week or so, but now I can hardly last a day. Noel and I always make a point to end our day on a good note. I would not wish MS on anyone, but it has given us a rare appreciation of every breath and taught us how to really enjoy the moment, and that is quite a nice way to live.

Noel replied instantly and said that he wanted shepherd's pie for dinner and added that he had an appointment with his neurologist the following week. He told me that he wanted to try one more blast of steroids. He said that I could accompany him if I wished and that I could ask his neurologist what he thought about LDN. Noel explained that if his neurologist gave it the go ahead then he would try it. I was delighted. He gave me a window and I was back in the game. All I had to do was convince Noel's neurologist of the merits of LDN.

I was excited and called Tia and Rachel. Being familiar with Noel, they knew that my excitement was premature, but kept encouraging me to continue. I spent days preparing for that appointment with Noel's neurologist. I called John from Town and Country Pharmacy to ask for his help. John assured me that he would send Noel's neurologist everything he had on LDN and he did. By the time the appointment came I was more than ready. I will never forget that consultation with Noel's neurologist in September 2002.

I dropped my children off with Tia and Rachel at Tia's house and I met Noel in the waiting room of the neurologist's office. I had a folder under my arm filled with papers which made Noel glare at me on arrival and question what on earth I was planning to do. I told him I was certain that his neurologist would prove difficult so I had to take a couple of print outs in case I forgot to say something. This made Noel very angry. He told me outright not to embarrass him by harassing his neurologist. I laughed nervously and assured him that I would be on my best behavior. Noel eyeballed me and told me that it was not a game. I assured him that a game was the last thing I would compare our situation to. Just then, Noel was called in and I followed. We both sat in the neurologist's office.

As always, the appointment started with the neurological exam. I am sure that this exam reveals something, but Noel literally staggered into the office with his cane (which he didn't have on his previous visit). However, because

Noel could still stretch out his arms and touch his nose it was deduced that there had been no change in him. Obviously, the tests are more thorough than I give them credit for, but I couldn't believe that it was decided that he had not progressed.

I was starting to twitch myself at this point, but I said nothing. The neurologist asked Noel what the problem was and Noel replied that he was feeling a bit weaker than usual and felt that he needed another blast of steroids. The neurologist proceeded to write the standard prescription and Noel started to get ready to leave. I asked politely if I could say something.

They both looked at each other and then they looked at me. I was tired, desperate, obsessed and even out of order because the neurologist did everything by the book and to step outside of that book leaves the guy open to all sorts of liability claims.

I said that I was delighted Noel could still touch his nose, but pointed out that I was concerned because he could no longer cut the grass, climb the stairs or get off the couch without falling over. I said that I was also concerned because he was taking a medication for Relapsing Remitting MS when it was clear he had Primary Progressive MS and I stated very clearly that Avonex was drastically failing him.

The neurologist asked me to describe Noel's decline. I gave a blow by blow account of his rapidly decreasing level of functionality. The neurologist genuinely appreciated the insight and suggested that perhaps Noel should come off Avonex and start a daily injection of Copaxone instead. Noel was not a bit pleased. He glared at me and a white rim started to form around his tightly clenched mouth. I continued.

I told the neurologist that Copaxone was also only recommended for Relapsing Remitting MS. I then showed him a number of printouts from the drug companies stating that their medications were all for Relapsing Remitting MS only. I even highlighted the printed probability of them working on that type of MS and the lists of side-effects they presented. I looked the neurologist in the eye and asked him if he honestly thought any of them were worth our while considering our circumstance. I said that our situation was desperate and that I wanted him to prescribe LDN for Noel. Then I asked him if he had read the literature forwarded by John Herr from Town and Country Pharmacy. He hadn't.

The neurologist sat down and asked me to take a seat. He told me that I was obviously under a great deal of stress and assured me that there were professional people who could help me work through my grief. Noel could not hold back any longer and apologized to his neurologist on my behalf. Noel glared at me and told me that I needed to speak to someone fast and work out my mental issues. I looked at them both calmly and agreed that it was quite possible that I did in fact need counseling. Without a doubt, I would have greatly benefited from intensive therapy. I mean, once again Noel's neurologist was simply going by the book, but I refused to accept that. I told them that I would look into therapy if it meant that they would just listen to me. I thanked them calmly for their concern for my mental health and proceeded.

When I finished the LDN theory, the neurologist raised his eyebrows at me and reminded me of all the MS meetings he attended. He told me that LDN had not gone through any scientific trial and if there was anything at all worth knowing about LDN then he would know about it. I then asked him outright if it could possibly do Noel any harm. He shrugged and said that he couldn't see what possible harm it could cause. I told him that at least we agreed on something and asked him to work with me. I asked him that seeing as we both agreed that it could do no harm, would he prescribe it. Noel was fit to kill me at this point. The neurologist thought about it for a brief moment and then wrote a script for 3 mg LDN. He also wrote a script for Copaxone and finished the one he started for steroids.

I have learned since then that it is common practice for neurologists to put their Primary Progressive MS patients on MS medicines that have only been tested on Relapsing Remitting MS. This is done because many neurologists feel that it is the best interest of the patient. I should also point out that many Primary Progressive MS'ers are very grateful for that.

Noel and I left the office in complete silence and drove home separately. I thought that the meeting went as well as could have been expected. We had the script so Noel could start LDN if he so wished.

I got home and Noel was irate. He was furious at me for telling his neurologist how to treat him. I knew that it was time to be quiet. Noel was very, very angry. For the rest of the day it was all picture and no sound in the Bradley house.

Chapter 16

"When we can't see eye to eye,
we can still see heart to heart."

Marge Lawler.

I remember the date of that appointment with Noel's neurologist because it was September 11th 2002. A good friend of ours lost her husband in the World Trade Center the year before and a gang of us from the Moms Group had planned to meet at the Nativity Church for the memorial service.

Late that evening Noel told me that he wanted to attend the mass. That meant I would have to stay home to put the children to bed. He planned to pick up his prescription for steroids when he was out and told me in no uncertain terms that I was never to get involved with his MS ever again. He was absolutely mortified at his neurologist's office. He said that he had no idea how far I was willing to take it. I said nothing because I had aggravated him enough and on top of my anger, I felt guilty for upsetting him so much. I promised him that I would never get involved again.

When I put the children to sleep I logged on to Goodshape's site to update the gang in cyberspace. I told them that I was going to back off all attempts to persuade Noel to try LDN because I felt like I was doing more harm than good. I silently wanted to kill Noel, but I didn't share that on the internet. The support from the Goodshape site was instant and sincere. They understood.

Noel arrived home after the memorial mass and to my amazement he was in great spirits. He even invited the Moms Group to come to our house. They all knew the pressure we were under and although I didn't feel like company at the time, they are always more than welcome in our home. They had become our family at this stage. I looked at Noel and told him that he had serious nerve to consider me crazy and asked him whatever happened to the angry guy who left the house earlier. He laughed and hugged me. He told me that he spent the mass thinking about everything.

Noel calmed down in church and like most people at rock bottom, he decided that it was time to pray for guidance. He apologized to me for implying to his neurologist that I was crazy. Everybody laughed and assured him jokingly that he was probably right. He told me that he would try LDN. He said that if I was that sure about it then maybe St. Anthony had a hand in it after all. He trusted that I had researched it as well as it seemed, and concluded that maybe it was worth a shot. I told him that it no longer bothered me what he did and said that he could take LDN or lump it because it was all the same to me.

At that point, Tia and Rachel thumped me. Rachel gave me quite a good whack on the arm. I laughed at their eye-bulging facial expressions and understood they were trying to tell me that I finally got what I wanted and to take it fast, so I somehow stopped being angry. Noel gave me the LDN prescription so I could get it filled in the morning. I took it and we called a truce. Noel made a pitcher of margaritas and we all hung out for a few hours and relaxed.

The following day, John compounded the LDN in Town and Country pharmacy in Ridgewood, and Noel started 3 mg LDN on September 12th 2002. Noel was still taking Avonex because he had just received a month's supply and he also started a course of steroids (prednisone) that night. I told Noel that he had to stop Avonex for LDN to work properly because Avonex suppresses the immune system whereas LDN boosts it. He looked at me bewildered, so I quickly added that the steroids probably weren't a good idea either. Noel said nothing.

That was the most difficult crossroads of our entire LDN journey. Noel's neurologist had told him that although Noel may have been doing poorly, he would have been a great deal worse off if he hadn't been taking Avonex. Copaxone is the only MS medication that doesn't work by suppressing the immune system so I explained to Noel that he could take Copaxone with LDN, but added that most of the people reporting success on LDN were taking LDN alone. I didn't want Noel to take Copaxone unless he absolutely had to because of the long list of scary side-effects. Noel was very nervous and rightly so. To take LDN, he had to go against what his neurologist thought best for him. I cannot express how difficult a decision that was for him and to be honest, I still cannot believe he went for it. I mean really, who would listen to their spouse over their neurologist? Who should?

Noel came up with a plan. He decided that he would try LDN on its own, but if he started to decline really rapidly then he would immediately add Copaxone to the protocol.

He hated a weekly injection and the thought of one daily was not very appealing. It was a very scary time, but we were united and that felt good. Noel stopped Avonex injections towards the end of September 2002 and replaced them with a nightly pill of LDN. He never started Copaxone.

In the midst of all of the craziness, I called my Aunt Annie to tell her that LDN may hold hope for Neilus and his Parkinson's. I also told Mom that it held tremendous hope for her breast cancer. It amazes me the different ways people react to LDN. With Noel I had to pump LDN, but with Neilus I had to deflate it. Neilus was willing to hop on the next plane out of Ireland to meet Dr. Bihari and see what the guy had to offer. Neilus was very easy to work with in comparison to Noel. I told Neilus not to get his hopes up too high, but also said that it was certainly worth investigating. Neilus instantly wanted to know everything and Annie told me to make an appointment with Dr. Bihari for Neilus. I called Dr. Bihari and made an appointment for Neilus for October 4th 2002.

Just as Noel was starting LDN, Mom, Dad, Annie and Neilus arrived at the airport. I went to meet them and immediately noticed that Neilus had progressed. In Irish tradition there was no point telling me or preparing me for that fact. A quick, short shock at the airport is considered better than weeks of worry. In keeping with traditions, I told Neilus that he never looked better. At this point I had read far too much about Parkinson's and that night I asked Annie if Neilus was taking any of the standard Parkinson's medications.

As with MS, there is no treatment to stop the progression of Parkinson's, but there are medications to control the symptoms. Such medications are not without some brutal side-effects. To make matters worse, Neilus had a hernia and his stomach was very sensitive to medication. Neilus could hardly tolerate an aspirin, not to mention the most common Parkinson's medication, Levadopa. I could tell that Annie was worried, but she hid it well. We were all worried because it was likely that Neilus would have to suffer Parkinson's without any medication because the chances of him being able to tolerate anything were very slim.

It was so nice to have the gang visit. I needed them and so did Noel. They are amazing people because of their ability to see good in everything. Neilus and Dad checked out our house and quickly started devising a plan to make it better. It needed a paint job and the back yard needed gutting. They were delighted that they would have something to do to pass the time. Mom and Annie promised to make it easy for them to get their work done by taking the kids to the mall daily. The kids adore their Grandparents. Of course they would, it is like Christmas everyday when they are around. Everyone was really happy.

I remember one night when we were going to bed Noel told me how much he admired my family. He said that he loved them because they understood life. I knew what he meant. Although he had only been on LDN for about two weeks or so, we had resumed our ability to be intimate again. I don't think that either of us will ever take that for granted in future.

Chapter 17

*"Two roads diverged in a wood, and I took the one less
traveled by, and that has made all the difference."*
Robert Frost

October 4th came and I was nervous. I was very
nervous, but in true Irish style, I completely hid it.
To be honest, I don't know what I was thinking that day because what we ended up doing made no sense whatsoever.
The appointment with Dr. Bihari was at 3:30 p.m..

Dad was eager to paint the whole downstairs of our
house that day and started preparing to paint as soon as he
woke up. Noel went to work as usual in the morning and I
logged on to the internet to print out the directions to Dr.
Bihari's office. Although the address seemed to be in a
reputable area of New York, I still had no idea what to expect. I was very aware that I had no real knowledge of Dr.
Bihari because I had not actually met him and all references

I had regarding his work came from one phone call and cyberspace.

I love Neilus and I really wanted the day to go well. So, being used to doctor appointments that lasted about twenty minutes, I decided that Mom, Annie and my three girls should accompany us. I thought that we could do something fun in New York together after the consultation. It seemed like a reasonable plan at the time. To make sure we arrived on time, I suggested we piled into the car at 2:00 p.m.. What a day lay ahead. Dad had his overalls on and paint brush ready on our departure so we waved goodbye to him and headed for New York. My dad is great. There is nothing he cannot do. He is smart too because there was no way he was going to join us in New York that day.

I knew the way up until we crossed the George Washington Bridge. As we were crossing I explained to the gang that I needed a navigator. Neilus assumed the position because Mom and Annie (also known as "the Grannies") who were in the backseats could not hear me with the want for a bathroom break among the children. Neilus quickly discovered that he forgot his reading glasses so the pair in the back shared theirs. Apparently, they all have the same prescription.

The party in the back meant I could not hear Neilus' directions, so we got lost. We laughed because we ended up in the slums of New York. We knew that New York was a grid and that makes it impossible to get truly lost, but time was becoming an issue. We honestly laughed so much that the children kept asking us what was so funny and the more they asked the more we laughed.

We finally found the address with about five minutes to spare. Annie decided that I should attend the consultation with Dr. Bihari and Neilus. I was very keen to do so and she knew that. I really wanted to meet Dr. Bihari and had many questions. I told the gang to sit tight in the car and added that we wouldn't be long. We would most likely be half an hour I told them, so I parked in front of the building.

Neilus and I entered 29 West 15th Street. We got into the elevator and on exit were greeted by Dr. Bihari's wife, Jacquie. She was very friendly. She took Neilus' details and proceeded to tell us that "Bernie" had no idea how to relax. She said that she was concerned for his health because he had no idea how to switch off from his work.

"Dr. Bihari is a workaholic!" she exclaimed.

Neilus can relate well to workaholics as he is the ultimate workaholic himself because he loves what he does. We both thought that Annic would have been able to relate well to Jacquie. I liked Jacquie. She had no issue expressing herself. I thought she was lovely.

Dr. Bihari called us in quite promptly. His office was by no means your typical doctor's office, nor was he your typical doctor. I felt like we were entering his living room. Dr. Bihari made us both feel instantly at home. I immediately scanned the area and liked the fact that he had pictures of his family surrounding him. His degrees and certificates, although many and present, were by no means the focus. Dr. Bihari looked to be about seventy, in good health and wore a suit that he was comfortable in. We sat on a very comfortable sofa-like piece of furniture and Dr. Bihari looked at Neilus and asked him what he did for a living. I instantly liked Dr. Bihari. It was apparent from the start that he cared, so I relaxed. I knew that Dr. Bihari asked that question to see if Neilus' Parkinson's was related to his profession, but I also knew that if Neilus liked to talk about anything, it was his work.

Neilus has a passion for boats. He spent his life building, buying, selling and dealing with boats. He is the type of guy who can wear a suit to convince the politicians to let him run the Island Ferryboat or a pair of overalls covered in grease to fix an engine. I always enjoy Neilus. He is a gentle giant and great with people. It was amusing to listen to him describe his accomplishments so modestly to Dr. Bihari, but he did tell the doctor everything he needed to know.

Neilus traveled a great deal, worked twelve hour days and often worked overnight in the shipyard in Downings, in Donegal. Neilus explained that although he was diagnosed with Parkinson's in 2001, he really had it since 1999. He said that it was slowly getting worse. At this time, his arm had a very obvious tremor and his facial expression was pretty blank. Neilus also had a mild tremor in his right leg and his gait was affected because his steps were shorter than average. Dr. Bihari examined Neilus and confirmed that he had Parkinson's. Apparently, Neilus had certain reflexes that were not working right and Dr. Bihari said the absence of such made the diagnosis easy. Then Dr. Bihari took a complete health history. I had been to many doctors through Noel, but I was impressed with how thorough Dr. Bihari was. I also could not believe how relaxed he was.

The cause of Parkinson's always bothered Neilus because nobody in our family ever had it and we can trace our family tree back for generations and generations. Dr. Bihari asked him to describe what was going on in his life when he first noticed the symptoms. Neilus explained his personal theory. He said that when the symptoms started it was during one of the most stressful periods of his life and he always wondered if it was the stress that triggered the disease. Dr. Bihari said that in his experience as a doctor he could not rule out stress as a major factor.

Dr. Bihari explained it like this. He said that we are all born with a particular set of genes that make us genetically susceptible to certain cancers and illnesses from birth. What struck him most in his profession was how common it was for people to contract cancer or some other illness a year or two after retirement in particular. Dr. Bihari said that he thought that after a stressful event, especially as we age, whatever it is that we are genetically predisposed to get, we will most like get. He explained that the stress may trigger a susceptible gene, but often it takes time for the symptoms to show. He said that he believed LDN could prevent many of those illnesses from occurring because many of the illnesses involve the immune system. In his experience, he explained again, that everyone with an auto-immune disease has low levels of endorphins and by taking LDN nightly this problem is rectified and the immune system becomes capable of functioning properly and keeps disease at bay. That was why he took LDN himself for the last ten years, he told us. He felt that LDN was helping him beat the odds of getting sick.

I asked him what made endorphin levels plummet. He said that he didn't know for sure, but was convinced that stress and aging were key factors. Dr. Bihari told us that once endorphin levels drop, they are not able to come back up on their own. He said that is what LDN is for. I asked him if there was a blood test to determine the exact state of Neilus' endorphins. He explained that there was one, but it was not your typical test and was not that straightforward. Blood needs to be drawn at the same time daily over a period of time to chart endorphin production properly. He said that he didn't feel that Neilus needed blood work because the testing he did on people in the early days of his discovery confirmed that all people with an autoimmune disease have low levels of endorphins. He was sure that Neilus would not turn out to be any different. Dr. Bihari was pretty sure that Parkinson's is an autoimmune disease.

Everything he said really did make sense. It made sense to a pair in dire need of a way to stop Parkinson's, at any rate. Neilus proceeded to ask Dr. Bihari about Parkinson's. Neilus asked him why he thought LDN would work for Parkinson's.

Parkinson's disease is a chronic progressive neurological disease that affects a small area of nerve cells in an area of the brain known as the substantia nigra. These cells normally produce dopamine, a chemical that transmits signals between areas in the brain that, when working normally, coordinate smooth and balanced muscle movement. Parkinson's disease causes these nerve cells to die, and as a result, body movements are affected. Dr. Bihari believed that in Parkinson's, the immune system attacks the substantia nigra. He said that was why he believed it is autoimmune and that was why he figured that LDN would work for Parkinson's. Although it was too early to say for sure how well LDN would work for Parkinson's, Dr. Bihari was convinced that it would stop it from progressing. He told Neilus about his three patients with Parkinson's who were on LDN for a year and were, by all accounts, proving his theory.

Dr. Bihari told Neilus that he was pretty sure that Neilus would not progress any further. How unbelievable is that? He said that he would have a clearer view of things in a year or so, but reiterated that it looked very promising. It was a great deal of information to take in and believe, but we did.

Neilus and I have many similar traits and one of those is our ability to get absorbed in something and completely forget about everything else. That day, we completely forgot about the gang in the car. We were nearly two hours into the appointment when we heard a car alarm on the street. I looked at my watch and thought I had better check on them.

I went out to the elevator and waited for it to arrive. My mind was racing. I could hardly take in all I had heard. I realized that if even a fraction of Dr. Bihari's theories were true then millions of families stood to be helped. I started to make a mental list of questions I needed to ask Dr. Bihari when I had the chance. Then I noticed that the elevator was taking a long time to arrive and I realized that I forgot to press the calling button. By the time I got downstairs, the car alarm was off. I opened the front door and could see the gang in the car laughing, so I quickly headed back upstairs.

I asked Dr. Bihari why he thought the medical community did not recognize the drug. He told me that he had been trying for years to get a clinical trial underway. He said that he desperately wanted a scientific clinical trial of LDN and AIDS. The main problem, he said, was that LDN is cheap. To get the drug FDA approved for AIDS or MS would cost a couple of million he said, and because the drug is cheap and already FDA approved at the higher dose, nobody in the U.S. would make a profit. He told me that he was more than eager to have his work scrutinized in the hope that LDN would reach the masses and gain scientific recognition. He said that his biggest concern was that he was getting on in years and that he may not be around long enough to see it all through. I asked him if he tried outside the U.S.. He said that he was trying to work with developing countries around the world with a view to LDN and AIDS. He explained that he had initiated a project for the developing world called The Developing Nations Project and that he started a foundation called the Foundation for Immunological Research in an effort to get things off the ground. He shared that he was not having a great deal of luck, as of yet, but he said that the internet was proving to be the tool that he was waiting for to help get the word out. Dr. Bihari added that he was willing to travel anywhere in the world to conduct a trial if a reputable body was willing to set one up. It was difficult not to like the guy.

I asked him if he remembered talking with me on the phone a while back. He said that he did and asked me what my husband decided to do. I told him that Noel had started LDN after a grueling appointment with his neurologist. I told him about the appointment and Dr. Bihari laughed, and so did I. I told him that Noel's neurologist really thought that I needed therapy.

I told Dr. Bihari that although Noel was taking LDN, he was not convinced that it would work. I explained that Noel had to play things safe and that he had to mentally prepare for the worst because then, if it happened, he would ready. Noel, I explained, would never think that LDN would stop his MS because that would make him too vulnerable. He would never leave himself so wide open. I, on the other hand, I explained, had no problem whatsoever believing that LDN would work and should his MS progress again I would deal with it then. For now, in my mind, Noel's MS was going to stop and we were all going to live happily ever after.

Dr. Bihari told me to explain to Noel that he should increase his dose to 4.5 mg LDN because over the years Dr. Bihari concluded that although 3 mg works for a lot of people, 4.5 mg works best for most. The optimum LDN dose that covers most bases is 4.5 mg. Dr. Bihari discovered this by accident. A patient of his who was taking 3 mg nightly, took two pills one night by mistake and woke up the next morning feeling better than ever. That incident encouraged Dr. Bihari to experiment with LDN dosage and eventually conclude that 4.5 mg works best for the majority of people. Naturally, there are exceptions to the rule, but Dr. Bihari's advice is to make sure that the dose is less than

10 mg to make sure that one doesn't block the opioid receptors for too long. If the receptors are blocked for too
long then endorphin production will not be tripled. More
LDN does not mean more endorphin production and better
results. Too much LDN, results in a lengthy opioid blockade, which results in less endorphin production and can result in disease progression, not retardation. Dr. Bihari
believes that as a general rule, people should start on 4.5
mg LDN and only experiment if problems emerge.

I asked Dr. Bihari about side-effects for Neilus and explained my concern that Neilus may not tolerate LDN. Dr.
Bihari told me that LDN is very easily tolerated. The most
common side-effects, he said, are vivid dreams and some
restless nights for a week or two, but nothing major. He
also assured me that LDN could be taken safely with any
other medication, except narcotics.

I asked if Neilus or Noel should wear a medical bracelet
in case they were in an accident. Dr. Bihari thought not. He
said that the dose is so low that it does not stay in the system long enough to be a serious medical threat. If Neilus
was in an accident and given narcotics for example, they
would not kill him. I told Dr. Bihari that my mom was in
the car and he remembered that she had breast cancer. I
asked him if I could make an appointment for her before
she flew back to Ireland. Jacquie checked his schedule, but
there was nothing available. He told me that it was clear to
him that she should be on LDN and offered to write her a
script. I was delighted. I wanted to put my entire family on
LDN immediately.

When he wrote the script for Neilus and Mom he
started on a third. It was for Noel. He gave it to me in case I
had trouble getting a renewal from Noel's neurologist. I
was so relieved because I was dreading another battle with
Noel's neurologist. We thanked Dr. Bihari and left. We

were speechless in the elevator. We felt wonderful. It was a great deal of hope to take in for one day.

We decided to head to Irmat's Pharmacy in NYC to fill the prescriptions right away. Dr. Bihari specifically recommended Irmats. We got to the car and I told the gang that we had to hurry because Irmats closed at six o'clock, which gave us less than ten minutes to find them. The children still needed a bathroom break and the Grannies were worn out singing "Wheels on the Bus" to keep them amused. They looked shattered, but happy.

We headed for Irmats. When I was in Irmats getting the prescription filled, a car alarm went off. This time I assumed that it was somebody else's alarm, so I took my time. When I got back to the car I discovered that it was my car alarm. The children were crying hysterically. Car alarms and elevators used to set them off all the time. Neilus was pacing outside the car and the Grannies looked numb. I tried to turn off the alarm, but I couldn't.

A passerby told us that The Empire State Building was responsible. Car alarms all over the city were going off uncontrollably. As we waited for about an hour and a half for AAA (American Automobile Association) to rescue us, many complete strangers tried to help us to turn it off. I love New York. I have no idea why anyone would think it unfriendly. I love the people. Finally, a guy succeeded in switching off the alarm. He lived locally and his name was Jarmane. He was so excited by his accomplishment that he jumped up and punched the air three times. He was a character and made us laugh. We thanked him for his help and headed for home.

I think that all of the passengers were relieved to reach the Jersey side of the George Washington Bridge because it had been a long day. We were all glad to get home. Dad had finished his paint job and the house looked great. He asked the girls if they had fun in New York. They told him that they had the best day ever and they meant it. That made the Grannies crack up laughing. I told him that we did have a great day and I really meant it too. We were all so relieved after the consultation with Dr. Bihari that I honestly don't think anything could have dampened our spirits.

Mom had a similar view of her cancer that Noel had of his MS. It was all in God's hands, so whether she took LDN or didn't take LDN, mattered very little to her. However, she knew what I had just experienced when trying to persuade Noel, so she decided to humor me on the basis that it could do her no harm. She refused to cause me any grief whatsoever. That night, October 4th 2002, Neilus, Mom and Noel started 4.5 mg LDN nightly.

Chapter 18

"When something important is going on, silence is a lie."
A.M. Rosenthal

I remember feeling delighted that evening. I was filled with hope. I was tired, but very happy. Annie asked me what she should expect. I told her that LDN is not a cure. Dr. Bihari's theory is that Neilus would not reach a point lower than his lowest point pre LDN. I told her to think of his worst possible day. I explained that that had to be the measuring stick. If he dipped below that point, then we would start to question it all, but until then I told her that I was prepared to believe Dr. Bihari. He was compassionate and genuine, and really believed what he said to be true. He was absolutely not a quack or a gangster.

The biggest question in my mind even back then, was how right was Dr. Bihari? I believed the stories in cyberspace and I had no doubt that he had discovered something big, but how big was always the question. I figured that only time would tell. We would just have to wait and see how effective LDN really was.

At first the improvements were stark. Noel really started to pull back very fast. It was incredible. Within six weeks his bladder had greatly improved and he stopped falling over. Although he still needed his cane around the house, he was able to take six or seven steps without it. There were definite improvements, but the most amazing thing for me was that the onslaught had finally stopped. Noel's MS had stopped progressing. Could the nightmare really be over? For the first time ever, I felt that his MS was under arrest. There is nothing better than the release from the onslaught of a progressive degenerative disease. As always, Noel remained calm. He didn't get overly excited because mentally he did not buy into it all. He couldn't afford to do that, but our family and friends could not believe the visible improvement in him. They were happy days.

Mom, Dad, Annie and Neilus flew back to Ireland in early November. Shortly after they left, my younger brother Kevin and his wife, Lisa, moved in with us because they were attempting a transfer to the U.S.. They stayed with us for about three months before returning to Ireland to settle. Sadly, the U.S. job market was stagnant due to September 11th. Still, it was nice to have the company for a while. By the time they arrived I think that Noel had reached his plateau. Some of the initial improvements faded, but his most recent symptoms pre LDN never returned. LDN reversed the most recent damage. Kevin deduced that Noel looked the same as he did in Ireland back in May. That was huge to me because I knew that Noel had slipped a great deal between May and September. For a while, MS went into the background and once again, life took over.

I kept in constant contact with Neilus and Annie. We

discarded tradition and agreed that our communication would always be open and honest. As time passed, it became obvious that Neilus' Parkinson's had also stopped progressing. He told me that he was doing better than ever. He was even able to weld again. Honestly, it was incredible.

Mom was more difficult to measure. She felt the same on LDN, as she did before she started it. She didn't notice any difference. I felt relieved that she was taking LDN and I stopped worrying before her routine check-ups.

All in all, things were great. Noel, Mom and Neilus were healthy again and thriving thanks to Dr. Bihari and LDN. Life was very good and was to remain so for quite some time. Thank God, we were given a break at last. It was a pleasure to ring in 2003.

It is odd, as I try to write the next part of this story that I should find it so difficult. Much time has passed since January 2003. Before I continue, I will share that word has leaked out among friends and family regarding my ambition to give a true account of my experiences with LDN and the reception is mixed. I suppose the bottom line is that my nearest and dearest, as always, are naturally trying to protect me. I fear that some feel like I am fighting a useless fight. I don't think so. My ambition with regard to this story is clear.

I want to see a large scale scientific trial for a cheap drug that holds great promise for millions. I don't expect or want anybody to have to take my word as gospel that the drug works. I don't want that responsibility. Instead, I want to see pressure put on a Government, University or Pharmaceutical Company to take the initiative to set up a trial. As the story unfolds it will become clear that I am not alone in this quest, far from it. Many people who have also seen or experienced first hand the implications of this medication feel an equal moral obligation to reach out to others.

But before I continue, I want to share one more thing.

I have to date, received many e-mails of gratitude from people all around the world who have started LDN and have experienced much benefit. When I read of references referring to my altruistic nature, it is important that I clarify. As I have written, I have three children. Since becoming a mother I relate much better to my own mother. My every breath is for them. In my mind, they are possibly genetically predisposed to acquire an autoimmune disorder. Should that happen, I want to challenge Dr. Bihari's theory today because if it is proven to be correct, then tomorrow's generation with autoimmune diseases will be treated much more effectively from the very start of their illness. Imagine taking your child to a neurologist and being told that he or she has MS or Crohn's, and then imagine the neurologist explaining that it used to be a big deal, but it isn't anymore. I know that I don't worry as much about the future health of my children because I know about LDN. I also know that people in my situation will appreciate the enormity of not having that weight on my shoulders anymore. But I want solid scientific proof so that I don't have to sound like I think I am a doctor when I talk about LDN to people who desperately need to hear about it. There lies a definite moral duty I cannot shake and believe me, I know that I am not a doctor, but I also know that you don't have to be that smart to figure out whether or not you or someone you love needs LDN. Sadly, most people just have to be desperate. I don't want anyone to feel as desperate as I did, when I know it could be prevented. As long as people know about LDN, I will utterly respect their decision as to whether or not they want to take it. As long as the world has heard about LDN, my job is done.

Today, most people with an autoimmune disorder are given steroids and antibiotics. There is no treatment, just symptom management. Often, there isn't even a name for sporadic, phantom symptoms stemming from a disturbed immune system. Millions of people are sick and don't even know why. They all need to hear about LDN. It is a fact that most immune based illnesses don't even have a name. I deeply feel for and empathize with all families afflicted with illness because I have lived the nightmare and that is why this is a story that I strongly feel has to be shared.

The promise LDN holds outweighs any personal embarrassment on my part. I want to see a large scale scientific clinical trial for LDN and MS. MS, because that is where the overwhelming testimonies lie. From there, who knows? So, I will continue, starting back at January 2003.

As January 2003 passed I became more and more convinced that LDN was working. Noel was, without question, stable. He no longer had to heave himself off the couch and for the first time in about ten years his feet were warm again. His complexion was also much better. I remember thinking that he just looked healthy. The biggest benefit was, of course, that the onslaught had stopped. Noel's spirits were, as always, good.

We didn't discuss LDN much at the time. Just as Noel never wanted to make MS his life, I knew that he would not want to make LDN his life either. He wanted to get on with life as best he could and so did I. I think that I actually forgot about MS for a while. I stopped reading the Goodshape message board and rarely researched anything on the internet. Life was very good.

I decided to take another trip back to Ireland in February 2003. The girls and I traveled ahead of Noel and, as always, he joined us for the second two weeks. This time he brought his own wheelchair and his journey went without incident. I really enjoyed that visit. It was the first time that we were without Noel and not worried about him having a relapse when we were gone. I believed that LDN would hold him and it did.

People in Ireland who had not seen Noel since May 2002 thought that he looked the same. That was a wonderful testimony for LDN because they missed his rapid decline. Also, it felt good to see Neilus thriving again. Like Noel, he looked healthy.

Unlike Noel, Neilus was very open about how good he felt on LDN. He was openly in shock that the drug was proving to be effective. Noel and Neilus decided to take one day at a time. They agreed that as with MS, the course in Parkinson's is unknown, but acknowledged that it looked very promising. For Noel to think that LDN was promising was a huge step forward.

Chapter 19

However long the night, the dawn will break.
African Proverb

W hen we settled back into New Jersey, my friend Paula, started to slip. At the time, she used the same neurologist as Noel. I consider Paula one of my closest friends and I desperately wanted her to take LDN because I believed it was working wonders for Noel. I thought that seeing as she had witnessed the effect LDN had on Noel, she would take LDN without question. It was not that straightforward.

I had to convince her as I did Noel and she proved to be just as stubborn with less reason. For a start, she refused all MS medications anyway so she didn't have to stop any drug in order to take it. Also, she had visible proof that it was working, not just stories from cyberspace. And, I assured her that Dr. Bihari was legitimate and genuine. I could not believe her resistance, but I would never judge or question it because I have no idea what it is actually like to have MS. I might have reacted exactly the same way myself.

Paula told me that the fact she had already refused MS medications automatically made her less likely to consider LDN. I never understood that, but I don't have to. Her MS was invisible to most people, but affecting her life. She was very tired every evening and her legs would give in sometimes when she climbed the stairs. Often, she was not able to climb the stairs when the day ended. Her legs were numb and tingling, but all of her symptoms always came and went. She had Relapsing Remitting MS and steroids always got her back on track whenever she slipped. Paula was not too keen to take LDN, but she decided to discuss the option with Noel.

Noel told her that if he were her, he would try it because it wouldn't do her any harm. He said that it helped him a little, but he didn't think that it helped him as much as everybody else said and claimed to see it did. He said that he still had no feeling in his legs, but was glad that at least he looked good to others. He could not have played it down more. Paula remained hesitant. I think that people with MS play mind games. I also think that they have to. Noel and Paula taught me that I will never fully understand the MS mindset. I think that Noel had to play down LDN to protect himself incase it failed and that Paula, at the time, found it difficult to believe she actually had MS.

Eventually, Paula went to see her neurologist and questioned him about LDN. He told her that he had one patient on LDN, but that as far as he knew it had no effect. The neurologist told her that he had discussed LDN with his colleagues and they decided it best not to prescribe it in future. His one patient was Noel who never went back to him because Dr. Bihari renewed his LDN script. Paula was aware of my meeting with her neurologist, so she decided it best not to acknowledge that she knew Noel and me.

Finally, Paula asked her neurologist if he would write her a prescription for LDN. She said that she had decided that she would like to try it. Her neurologist refused to write her a prescription for LDN and told her that she should seriously consider the shots. Paula refused the shots and left his office with a blast of steroids.

A couple of weeks passed. I called to Paula's house. Her symptoms were still bothering her. I told her that it was time she met with Dr. Bihari. She was still on the fence, but I put the phone in her hand and told her to make an appointment because enough was enough. She called and made an appointment. Paula and her husband met Dr. Bihari on March 8th 2003. Everybody I know who has met with Dr. Bihari has a story and I laughed out loud when I heard theirs.

Paula said that she was taken aback when she first met Dr. Bihari. He had had a recent hip operation and needed a cane to get around. She thought that he looked like death and could not believe that I didn't prepare her for the shock. I laughed because when I met him in October he looked like a healthy seventy-year-old to me. Although he was on LDN for ten years, I would agree that he wasn't exactly a poster child for it, but still, he was healthy. I also laughed when I imagined Jacquie scolding him for getting back to work so soon after surgery because I knew that his workaholic tendency bothered her. I respected and liked Dr. Bihari even more for working after surgery. It proved his dedication and belief in what he was doing.

Paula started LDN in the middle of March 2003. She started with the same mindset as Noel. She refused to believe that her MS would not progress. It was too dangerous for her to think like that. She tried LDN because it was reported to have no side-effects, was cheap and over-all she deduced that the promises outweighed the risks. I was glad that her insurance covered her consult with Dr. Bihari, so it wasn't a costly venture by any means.

Initially, Paula felt wonderful on LDN. She could not believe how great she felt and I was ecstatically happy for her. She had a great deal more energy and could not wait to tell her neurologist her success story. Then the unthinkable happened.

In July 2003, Paula started to relapse when taking LDN. I did not understand how that was possible because, at that time, I had never heard of anybody experience a relapse when taking LDN. All of her old symptoms came back with a vengeance. She did not experience anything brand-new, but her symptoms became more severe than she ever remembered. I also remember noticing that she developed foot drop and her ability to stand for any period of time had greatly diminished. That was a very scary time.

Paula seemed to be proving that the LDN theory was not true and was ready to pack it in. One day, during her re-lapse she called to my house and phoned Dr. Bihari to tell him what was happening to her. He told her to eat three bars of chocolate a day for the next three days. She hung up and looked at me, as if to say, "Why on earth do I ever lis-ten to you?" We looked at each other in disbelief and for the first time ever I began to wonder if Dr. Bihari was a quack because his advice sounded crazy. I decided that I had to investigate thoroughly.

My mind went back to the consult with Neilus. My gut still believed Dr. Bihari. I had already thoroughly checked out his credentials and judged his character to be honest. Growing up in the hotel business, I like to think, taught me how to read people quite well. Whether or not I had to be-lieve in Dr. Bihari for sanity I don't know, but I do know that I was not prepared to give up on LDN right away.

I remembered that Dr. Bihari said that LDN would only reverse the last three months of MS scarring on the spinal cord or brain for the lucky people and that all old scars would remain. Also, I remembered that he said that in times of personal stress or infection (fever, flu, etc.) the old scars might flare up, causing a reoccurrence of old symptoms, but he firmly believed that no new symptoms would develop. Paula did not experience any brand-new symptoms so I began to think that maybe the theory was still true. She didn't seem stressed though and she didn't look like she was running an infection, but something was clearly not right. It wasn't clear what was causing her olds scars to flare up.

I logged onto the Goodshape site and started to investigate. I posted two questions. I asked if any of them were aware of anybody who had relapsed while on LDN and I explained Paula's situation. Then I asked what chocolate had to do with LDN. The replies were most helpful and explained a great deal.

They told me that it was quite common for old symptoms to return in full force shortly after starting LDN. Some considered this a good sign and referred to it as a healing crisis. Paula didn't fall into this category because initially she was doing better than ever. She started to slip out of the blue, after initial improvement, so it could not have been a healing crisis.

Then a woman named Angelina spotted the problem. She convinced me that Paula was probably suffering from invisible Candida, a simple yeast infection, as a result of her steroid use pre LDN. Angelina had suffered similar infections and found LDN to be less effective when she had a yeast infection. She then told me about a simple test that my friend could perform to confirm whether or not her yeast levels were too high. Paula thought that if she was running a yeast infection she would know about it, but to humor me she took the test. I was actually happy when the test revealed that her yeast levels were very high.

A couple of days later Paula's mouth broke out in sores. Without question, she had a yeast infection. She addressed the infection, but lost confidence in LDN. She was not convinced that something so simple would set off all of her symptoms. She was also planning a trip to Disney with her family so she called her neurologist and began a course of steroids to get by.

It is January 2009 now and Paula has not taken steroids since July 2003 and remains on LDN despite a rocky start. That initial setback, understandably, left her more than cautious. I thank God that she is doing wonderful on LDN. She works five days a week, is an active community member and a wonderful mother. I don't think her daughters even know that their mother has MS. I am certain it does not affect their family life in any way. Her MS remains invisible to everyone. I often look at Paula playing with her kids and quietly say to myself, "Thank you God." She looks so good that sometimes I cannot help but wish that Noel found LDN when he was at Paula's stage of the disease.

Like everyone else I know on LDN, when Paula is stressed or running an infection, her old symptoms flare up, but she has not experienced any brand-new symptoms. Her MS has not progressed. I watch her like a hawk and cannot detect even slight foot drop anymore. Although she does not fully believe in LDN, she will not stop taking it, but remains mentally prepared for progression and more relapses.

The Goodshape board also educated me on chocolate and LDN. Many told me that they found it beneficial during times of stress. It turns out that there is an amino acid called DL Phenylalanine in chocolate which slows the breakdown of endorphins during the day. Dr. Bihari believes this works well with LDN because it helps to keep endorphin levels higher, for longer, daily. It helps to prolong the LDN effect. Many people on the board had chocolate allergies so knew to take the capsule supplement from any vitamin store instead. Some said that it worked wonders and others said that it didn't.

I have since spoken to Dr. Bihari about this and he now recommends the supplement instead of chocolate. He recommends 500 mg DL Phenylalanine in the morning and afternoon in times of stress or infection to help boost the LDN effect.

Noel, Neilus and Paula completely convinced me that Dr. Bihari had discovered something huge. Although they could not mentally buy into it all, watching them was proof enough for me.

In April 2004, Noel was taking LDN for about nine months with no progression. He went to see his neurologist, but I didn't go. I wasn't invited. After the neurological exam it was decided that Noel was the same as before and his neurologist advised him to keep on doing whatever he was doing.

Paula has since been to see the same neurologist and tried to convince him that she thought LDN was helping her, but he assured her that it wasn't. He told her that if she remained relapse free for about three years then maybe he would start to look into it. Paula did remain relapse free for over three years, but in the meantime, changed her neurologist.

Their ex-neurologist was an excellent neurologist, by the way. He was a typical neurologist who went strictly by the book and firmly believed that he knew everything there was to know about MS.

Chapter 20

*"Be kinder than necessary because everyone
you meet is fighting some kind of battle."*

Anonymous

One day in the middle of the summer of 2003, I decided it was time to let people know about LDN. I hated to think of all the people with MS or any autoimmune disorder who were progressing when there was something so simple available to help them.

Since that time I have met many people who have truly amazed and inspired me. I have also learned much about how the world works. It has been an interesting journey, to say the least.

Ireland seemed like the most sensible place to start because the Irish Government pays for all of the costly MS medications there. I began to investigate how many people in Ireland were taking LDN. I was already aware of one lady, Mauka, whom I spoke with on the Goodshape message board back in September 2002.

During that period in 2002 when Noel's job was insecure, I was trying to figure out how he would obtain LDN if we had to move back to Ireland. This was before I met Dr. Bihari and discovered that Irmats Pharmacy in New York and Skips Pharmacy in Florida ship worldwide. Mauka was incredibly helpful. She heard about LDN through the Goodshape site and was based in Wicklow. Her neurologist was based in St. Vincent's in Dublin. She told me that her neurologist was more than skeptical about prescribing LDN and it took a great deal of convincing on her part to actually get the prescription. On top of that, she then had to find somewhere in Ireland to compound LDN.

In America, most compounding pharmacies pack 4.5 mg of pure Naltrexone powder into a capsule and because it is such a minute amount, they need to pad the capsule with some sort of inert substance, called a filler. The most important requirement when compounding LDN is that the filler used to pad the capsule ensures the fast release of the drug into the body. Although the expertise was available in Ireland at this time, the technology to make 4.5 mg LDN capsules was not.

Liquid LDN also ensures the fast release of Naltrexone into the body. People on the Goodshape board who were finding it difficult to get a prescription from their neurologist or doctor were legally importing 50 mg Naltrexone tablets, without a prescription, from Mexico and home brewing. They would add 50 ml of distilled water to one 50 mg tablet, shake it, let it dissolve and using a dropper, drink 4.5 ml nightly. People who homebrewed their own liquid LDN were reporting great success. Many preferred to homebrew for a number of reasons: It ruled out compounding errors, it was even cheaper than the capsules and they could adjust their dose very easily until they found what dose worked best for them. Others did not like this method because a 50 mg Naltrexone pill weighs about 315 mg, meaning it contains 265 mg of filler and unlike Naltrexone, the filler is not soluble, so homemade liquid LDN is a little lumpy, has a bitter taste and is not as scientifically accurate as a compounding pharmacy.

I should point out that the patents held by Dr. Bihari and Dr. Zagon that I mentioned earlier, are *use patents*. This recognizes that there had been a patent for Naltrexone years ago (which is long gone), but establishes their rights in the U.S. to these discoveries of special uses for Naltrexone in a low dose. However, no big pharma is willing to kick in tens of millions of dollars to run trials for FDA approval for these special uses because anyone is able to buy 50 mg Naltrexone and dilute it for pennies to make many doses of LDN.

In Ireland, a pharmacy on Lower Lesson Street in Dublin, had a pharmacist named Ann who made up the LDN prescription for Mauka in a solution that stayed fresh for two weeks. Mauka received her LDN by post every two weeks in Wicklow from Dublin. Also, the Health Board for the Wicklow area covered the cost of Mauka's LDN under the Long Term Illness program. Mauka was delighted to have found LDN. Like everyone else with whom I was in contact at the time, she was stable. My last contact with her was in October 2003. She had just gone for her annual appointment with her neurologist and he detected no deterioration in her condition for the year she was on LDN. But better than that, she felt great within herself. She knew that she had not progressed and had no desire to ever stop taking LDN. As far as I know, Mauka was the first person in Ireland to take LDN. In July 2003, she was the only person besides Mom and Neilus, I could find in Ireland on LDN.

Chapter 21

"Greatness is a road leading towards the unknown."
Charles de Gaulle

I searched around a little more to try to find out if there were other people in Ireland taking LDN and when I could not find any, I decided to check out Britain. I came across a doctor in Wales named Dr. Robert Lawrence. He was easy to find because he had his own website with all of his information. He had MS himself and started taking LDN after reading about Dr. Bihari's work on Goodshape's site. He was so impressed with the results that he started to prescribe LDN for MS patients.

Initially, Dr. Lawrence imported LDN from the U.S. for his patients, until Martindale Pharmaceuticals in the UK started to supply him. The LDN movement was much more advanced in Britain than in Ireland thanks to the efforts of Dr. Lawrence. As in the US, people with MS all over Britain were reporting wonderful success stories on LDN on the internet. What was most remarkable was that LDN did seem to work for everyone, to a degree. LDN was working across the board.

I decided that I wanted everyone in Ireland to hear about LDN, so I started with the people I knew needed to hear about it yesterday. I phoned Dr. Muriel first. I will always be grateful to her for the hope she gave me in 1998 when I was at my lowest point. I explained the whole LDN theory to her and told her how well it was working for Noel. She told me that she would investigate and asked me to inform the top neurologist in Dublin. I knew that she was referring to Mauka's neurologist. I told her that he was already aware of it and even had one patient taking LDN, but she had to fight for her prescription. I told her that he did not want it known that he knew about LDN because LDN was not clinically trialed for use with MS. I suppose he feared people might consider him a quack or the medical board might threaten his medical license for acting outside of the book.

The years had made Dr. Muriel skeptical of miracle treatments for MS and I certainly did not blame her. Although delighted that LDN was working for Noel, she decided, in the end, that she would stick with conventional thinking. She told me that the shots were helping her. I completely respected her decision and felt good that at least she was now aware of LDN, should she need it in the future. My job was done.

Then I phoned Alma, the sister of my childhood friend, Coirle. Her husband, Robert, was doing quite poorly at the time. On top of MS, he was also starting a battle with another autoimmune illness, sarcoidosis. He was taking a weekly shot of Avonex, but they did not feel like it was helping him. I told Alma all about LDN. I told her that I knew that it sounded too good to be true, but she had to convince Robert of its merits if he was to have any chance of winning the fight. I told her that LDN would also help his sarcoidosis. I explained how difficult it was for me to convince Noel, but assured her that it was worth it. Alma was very grateful for the information and assured me that she would pass it all on to her husband and told me that she felt very confident that Robert would thoroughly investigate.

At this point in his life Robert was very tired in the evenings and he could never get enough sleep. No matter how much he slept, he never felt rested. He suffered serious joint pain too. At times he also used a cane for support. His quality of life was greatly impaired which naturally affected his wife and their two young children. Robert was also on a lot of medications, at the time, to deal with his symptoms. Alma told Robert all about LDN and Robert, as she predicted, thoroughly investigated everything on the internet immediately. He didn't waste one second.

In early July, Robert went to see his neurologist in Galway. His neurologist could see that Avonex did not seem to be doing Robert any favors and suggested that Robert should discontinue the shots. Robert told him that he was thinking of trying LDN. Robert's neurologist was political in his reply. He played it safe. He pointed out that there were no formal trials to back up anecdotal testimonies on the internet and added that as far as he knew, LDN was not available in Ireland. Robert said that that Dr. Lawrence in Wales could supply him.

The neurologist basically told Robert that if he wanted to go for it to do so, he was not going to try to stop him. He remained neutral which could be perceived as somewhat supportive. Shortly after that consult, Robert spoke with Dr. Lawrence on the phone and sent him his medical notes.

Robert started 3.5 mg LDN nightly in the middle of July 2003. He moved up to 4 mg towards the end of July.

Robert and Alma could not believe the effect LDN had on him. It was life changing. They thought it nothing short of a miracle. The first thing Robert noticed was that his joint pain disappeared. Then his energy levels soared and his over all general well being greatly improved. He no longer needed a selection of medications or a cane. LDN fixed all of his health problems. It was unbelievable.

Robert could not believe that the world didn't know about this tiny simple pill. He felt a strong moral obligation to let as many people as possible know about it so he immediately started to spread the word. Robert has since been interviewed many times. He is highly intelligent and an excellent storyteller and people could not help but listen to him. I liked the story about his trip to Valentia, in County Kerry, because it was tangible and powerful testimony for LDN

A month before Robert started on LDN he went on a business trip from Galway to Carlow. A work colleague drove him there and back, but it still took Robert three days to recover from the trip. Then, about a month after going on LDN he had a business meeting to attend in Valentia, County Kerry. He drove the five hour trip himself, attended a four hour meeting and drove back that same day himself. The following morning he went to work feeling fine. There was no recovery period required.

Then, shortly after that, his LDN supply got stuck in the post. He had to go seven days without it. Within those seven days his fatigue returned and he started to need his stick again. Once he resumed LDN, the symptoms disappeared as before. It is important to point out that it was a difficult decision for Robert to come off Avonex and go on LDN. As with Noel, it was a personal risk that he decided to take. To date, it is a risk that thousands of people have taken because they felt the standard MS medications did not work for them.

The more I talked with people during the summer of 2003, the clearer it became that LDN needed a scientific clinical trial so that people who wanted to try it would not feel as if they were gambling with their lives. I wanted to remove the fear from taking a chance on LDN. At the time, I didn't know how to approach the whole issue of a trial, but I knew that the first stage had to be getting the word out.

I figured that the best place to start was with the MS Societies. I thought that once they heard about LDN they would do everything in their power to get scientific recognition for LDN and help get it to the people who really needed it. There are many people with MS who take no medications at all, people who refuse the shots because of the nasty side-effects, but might consider LDN if they knew about it. I felt that they had a right to know about LDN and at least make up their own mind as to whether or not they wanted to try it. It was frustrating to feel that I knew something that everybody else should know.

The MS Ireland website has been changed since the summer of 2003, but they used to have a letters section to which I wrote a letter about Noel and LDN. I made it clear that the drug needed a scientific trial, but emphasized that it held tremendous hope, was cheap and had no side-effects. I checked the letters page of the website the following morning to see if I could view it, but it was not there. So, I wrote the letter again, but it never appeared on the website. I tried once more and when it never surfaced, I figured that I was being blocked. MS Ireland did not want me to tell the LDN story and that annoyed me.

I decided to investigate more. I noticed that it was the

policy of MS Ireland not to give advice on therapies that were not clinically proven. I respected that, but this was a letters page. This was me telling my story, not MS Ireland pumping LDN. I was simply telling a story in the hope that people could investigate and make up their own minds.

I read some of the other letters. Some spoke of bee stings and others mentioned a particular diet. These were not clinically proven, but yet were opinions that MS Ireland deemed okay to share. I appreciated reading the experiences of people on bee stings and diets, but it made me angry that I was not allowed to talk about LDN. I decided to dig deeper.

Then I learned that MS Ireland were practically completely financially dependant on the drug companies pumping out the expensive MS medications. How wrong is that? If the drug companies want to help people with MS then it should be made very clear, almost in the naming of the society, where the financial interests of the society rest. For example, why not call MS Ireland, Biogen's MS Ireland if it is true that they have indirect control. That way people could directly applaud Biogen for all the good work that they do to help people with MS. It would also avoid any potential confusion regarding possible conflict of interest when discussing other drugs, such as LDN, for MS. MS Ireland weren't going out of their way to sabotage LDN, they simply didn't want to know anything about it or let anyone else know anything about it through them.

I knew some people who worked in MS society branches around Ireland and I knew that they were good people. I knew that their hearts wanted the best for people with MS, despite the politics of the society. In general, most people who work for MS societies are directly affected by MS. Either they actually have the disease or a loved one has or did. MS is personal to them, so I knew

146

that many would listen. I often wonder how much more some neurologists would listen to the LDN theory if MS was personal to them. I would never wish MS to be personal for anybody, but I know that it makes all the difference in the world.

At that time, the MS Ireland website had a list of every single MS branch in Ireland. It didn't just list the regional head offices. It listed every branch in every nook and cranny of the country. There were thirty-nine in total. They even listed the names and phone numbers of the chairperson and secretary of each branch. Also, they had profiles of people with MS living in Ireland with their e-mail address attached. They certainly supplied me with a gold mine of information.

One afternoon that summer, when the children were resting, I started at the top of the phone list. My first phone call was to the Athlone branch where I spoke with Eileen. Every phone call I made turned into a lengthy one because not one office had ever even heard of LDN. I averaged about a call or two a day for the next while. It amazed me how quick the people were to share their personal MS nightmares. Eileen told me that she had a mild form of MS and that she considered herself very lucky. In the Ballina Branch, Mary had MS and was in wheelchair; in Bandon, Padraic's wife had MS for fifteen years; in Bray, Helen's husband was in a wheelchair; in Sligo, Kathleen's husband was bedridden with MS; in Letterkenny, John was battling MS and in Galway, Aidan's wife was also suffering. The list went on and on. It was harrowing. I cannot express how wonderful every representative from each branch was. Many were inspirational in how they dealt with MS or cared for a loved one. They were passionate and I could really relate. Many apologized on behalf of MS Ireland when I told them that my letter was blocked. Others said that they were saddened and shocked. Some took my e-mail address and phone number and promised that they would start to distribute LDN information to the public immediately.

Shortly after my phone calls, I started getting quite a lot of e-mail from people inquiring about LDN. I replied to all of them. I also personally e-mailed seventy-two people in Ireland who had their e-mail address openly available on the MS Ireland website. I was busy, but driven. Word about LDN was getting out all around Ireland and it was exciting. People were listening, they were really listening.

Many went straight to Dr. Lawrence in Wales and started LDN almost immediately and reported back tales of success and sincere gratitude. Many of the e-mails contained passionate stories that made a lump form in throat. It was incredible. I particularly remember a young guy from Galway, named Fergal Hughes, who desperately wanted to buy me a drink because he was going to climb Craogh Patrick since starting LDN. Fergal did climb Craogh Patrick. Then he married a lovely lady named Lisa and had a couple of babies. The last time we spoke, he was on LDN for four years with no progression and living happily ever after. I look forward to having that drink with him.

There were others who were hesitant and fearful and chose not to try LDN, but still appreciated the knowledge. I didn't receive any negative feedback. It was all very positive. I got to know a great deal of people that summer and I will never forget them. I am sure I will meet many face to face during future trips home. The best thing about all of it was that as people read about LDN and tried it, they also felt obligated to tell others. I loved the snowball effect.

In October 2003, The Sunday Business Post printed an article about LDN thanks to pressure from Robert. LDN was finally hitting the mainstream media and I, like many others at this stage, felt it was imperative to push for a trial.

MS experimental drug "could save state millions of Euro"

05/10/03 00:00

By Simon Carswell

A handful of multiple sclerosis (MS) sufferers in Ireland have switched to a new medication that costs just 4 per cent of the price of the drug commonly used to treat the disease.

Most of the 6,000 MS patients in the state use a drug called Beta Interferon. However, about a dozen Irish MS sufferers have switched to a drug called Low Dose Naltrexone (LDN), which boosts the immune system and is used to treat HIV/Aids and cancer.

A year's supply of Beta Interferon for an MS sufferer costs the state about €12,000, compared to €480 a year for LDN. Most Irish patients buy LDN from Dr. Robert Lawrence, a GP based in Wales who is himself an MS sufferer.

Dr. Lawrence said he has supplied the drug to about a dozen patients in Ireland, mostly in the west. The drug is approved by the FDA in the US, but no clinical trials have been carried out on it in Ireland or Britain. He said he explains this to patients before selling them the drug. "I explain when I introduce it to people that what they are using is experimental and that no trials have been carried out on it and that people must accept it as such," said Lawrence.

One MS sufferer, a businessman from Co Galway, said he switched from Beta Interferon to LDN in early August and since then has experienced "a dramatic difference" in health.

"It got rid of my fatigue and my joint pain, and also removed weakness in my lower limbs," he said. "I can now

work a full day and enjoy more time with my children, and life in general."

He urged the Department of Health to fund clinical trials and research of LDN, as it could save the state millions of euro every year.

Lawrence said he imports LDN from New York for resale in Britain and Ireland.

"The only reason I can imagine why no further research or investigation has been done is that, because the drug is so relatively cheap, no drug company is interested in producing it or supporting the trials that will get it accepted as an approved treatment for MS. There is simply no potential for significant profit," he said.

Maura McKeon, spokeswoman for the Multiple Sclerosis Society of Ireland, said: "Until trials are carried out on it, we cannot advise people to try this particular product. Up to now, we have received only anecdotal evidence of its effects."

Things were finally starting to happen and that felt good. I was delighted that Noel was still doing great, as was Neilus, my friend Paula, Robert and Goodshape's wife, Polly. The official LDN website was expanding rapidly and even started its own message board where people gathered to share their personal LDN experiences and encourage each other. Other message boards dedicated to LDN also started to appear on the internet. The word was spreading like wildfire.

Lifetime friendships and bonds formed during that period. Dr. Skip Lenz, a Floridian compounding pharmacist by trade and humanitarian by nature, posted the following on the LDN website:

From: Dr. Skip [Skip's Pharmacy, Boca Raton, FL]
Re: Naltrexone

Date: Thu Oct 23 18:21:35 2003

As I have said before, if I had MS, the only drug that I would absolutely be taking is LDN. I wouldn't care what it took, or who I had to insult. In four years of dispensing LDN, with over 10,000 patient months, I have heard of only three cases of exacerbation. I am waiting for our new resident to come in and I will have exact numbers, but this is truly a no-brainer. I would find some one to prescribe it no matter the cost or effort.

Dr. Skip

In April 2006, Dr. Skip spoke at the second LDN annual conference in Bethesda, Maryland. I raised my hand and asked him a question.

"Dr. Skip, what are your thoughts on taking LDN to prevent illness?"

"You are not asking me the right question Mary."

"What?"

"You should ask me if *I* take LDN to prevent illness."

"Do you?"

"Yes."

The last time I counted, Dr. Skip had 15,000 patients on LDN and was shipping the drug worldwide. His pharmacy distributes LDN at the lowest possible cost because underneath his beard and passionate nature lies an altruistic spirit. He sponsors, attends and speaks at every LDN conference and his lovely wife Cyndi and their son Adam, actually film every conference and distribute the DVD's at cost value or less around the world every year. I love the Lenz family. Dr. Skip is worth googling.

Getting back to 2003: As the first LDN snowball continued to roll, my eldest daughter, Annie, started school in

New Jersey, in September 2003. I met her teacher, Rosemary Konde, and it is a meeting I will share because it had a deep and probably everlasting effect on me.

Chapter 22

"Many people come into our lives and quietly go,
Others stay for just a little while longer
And leave footprints on our hearts;
And we are never the same again."

Anonymous

M y maternal Grandmother was a wonderful storyteller. When I was a child I used to stay up all
night long listening to her ghost stories. Sometimes my
mother would pretend-yell at us in the middle of the night,
and to get us out of trouble, Grandma would tell me happy
stories about real life angels she met here on earth. She was
convinced that at some point in time we are all a guardian
angel to somebody, whether we know it or not. I loved her
stories, but never, ever, believed one word. She was highly
intelligent and never left out any detail, so believe me, her
stories were very real, but I never believed them. Then, I

met Rosemary Konde. I know if I was told that I had an hour left to live I would include her in my thoughts. Grandma was right. Angels do exist on earth.

Rosemary was in a huge, tastefully and colorfully decorated classroom with her class of awkward five-year-olds on the floor around her. She sat on a rocking chair and wore a pair of eyeglasses on the tip of her nose. From a distance, I estimated that she was sixty or so, but up- close she was obviously only in her very early fifties. She had such a pleasant countenance and eyes that just looked at things right. As soon as I laid eyes on her, I felt as if I had known her all of my life. I was immediately drawn, like never before or since.

Like all of the other moms of her class, I believed that Annie Kate could not have landed a better kindergarten teacher and that was important to me, but beyond that, I felt a strong connection with Rosemary before I even spoke with her. I didn't acknowledge the connection, but I did sign up to help with class parties, and made a note of Rosemary's e-mail address to coordinate such events.

I shared my affection for Rosemary with Tia and we agreed it best that I kept my distance, to let the woman get on with her job. To tell her that she was remarkable, apart from making strained conversation, sounded false and crazy even, so we laughed about it. Often, when I would visit Tia, she would ask me how "Rosie" was doing and I would show her Annie's schoolwork and tease Tia that she was wasting her money sending her children to private school. Like every meeting I ever had with Tia, it was light and fun. We laughed all the time.

Then, around Thanksgiving, which is late November, I e-mailed all of my contacts in Ireland to inform them that I had written to Pat Kenny, a popular talk show host in Ireland. I was eager to get Dr. Bihari on Irish TV and was convinced that Pat Kenny would jump at the opportunity. I called Dr. Bihari before I sent the letter and was amazed that he was willing to travel to Ireland to help get the word out. As soon as I sent the e-mail I noticed that I included Rosemary by accident. I couldn't believe it. The last thing in the world I wanted was to divulge my LDN obsession with "Rosie."

Like every year back then, Tia and I met at 5:00 a.m. on the Friday after Thanksgiving to shop in the sales. We used to do all of our Santa shopping in one day. That Friday morning, when we were standing in line outside Toys R Us, I told Tia of my e-mail error. Tia laughed out loud because it was funny. We both laughed.

We were also laughing at the time because we just figured out why we were first in line. The store didn't open until 7:00 a.m.. We couldn't believe how wrong we got the time and how many other people were there on purpose. The TV crews were setting up and we laughed at the thought of the Moms Group seeing us on TV outside the store. As a group of young Moms we were unique because one of us was always in the midst of some calamity.

That Thanksgiving, I asked Tia what I should do about "Rosie" and we were torn as to whether or not I should pretend I didn't notice my e-mail error or own up to it. I decided to explain the LDN story to Rosemary in a follow up e-mail. I explained that I feared a plea for sanity would only confirm madness because I understood that the story was difficult for many people to believe due to the absence of a proper clinical trial. I knew that some people thought that I had to believe in LDN because I could not face the reality of MS. I also knew that that was not the case.

Rosemary replied to my second e-mail and I could hardly believe her reply. If you believe in coincidence it was a classic. As I mentioned earlier, I don't believe in coincidence. I am afraid to believe in coincidence out of fear I will miss a miracle. I like to think that everything happens for a reason.

Rosemary explained that a line from my e-mail that struck her was that Dr. Bihari claimed that all autoimmune diseases would respond to LDN. She said that she was absent from school that Wednesday because she was at the hospital with her twenty-six-year-old daughter, Kate, who needed her third surgery for nasal polyps and deviated septum. She explained that Kate was what is known as a Samters Triad patient, a condition which causes the patient to suffer from asthma, an intolerance to aspirin and severe nasal polyps. She described Kate as having no energy with a perpetual cold and no sense of smell and hence appetite. Then, she said that she believed that Samters was an autoimmune disease.

Rosemary believed that in Samters, the immune system attacks the nasal passages. She had already spent hours on the websites reading about Dr. Bihari and LDN in the hope that it would be helpful to Kate and she planned to bring it all to Kate's attention as soon as possible. By all accounts, Rosemary was delighted to have received the information. She was very glad of my mistake.

Rosemary presented the information to Kate and like her mom, Kate cut to the chase and could see that LDN could potentially help her. I instantly liked Kate. She was a fighter with great spirit and wit. I think that Kate and Rosemary kept their expectations realistic and thought LDN was worth a try seeing as it had no side-effects. Kate realized that she had little to lose and much to possibly gain by trying it. She took all of the information to her ENT (ear, nose and throat) doctor in early December 2003 and as expected he had never heard of LDN and did not want to prescribe it.

Kate immediately called Dr. Bihari. To her amazement, he spoke with her for about twenty-five minutes on the phone and she made an appointment to see him on Friday December 12th. Her mom, dad and husband attended the consult with her. I could not wait to hear how her appointment went and eagerly awaited the report. It was a good one.

Kate and her family were very impressed with Dr. Bihari. They thought him humble considering his accomplishments. Their appointment lasted about two hours. Dr. Bihari said that he had not seen a case like Kate's in thirty years and that her type of immune disease was very rare. He pointed out that in addition to the "big and famous" immune diseases such as MS, he believed that there are hundreds of other rare diseases, such as samters that get very little interest by the medical community because of their low rate of incidence in the population. Dr. Bihari questioned Kate very thoroughly as to her medical history, asthma, allergies, polyps, surgeries and medications. Then, he did a thorough questioning about her family's medical history. He was interested to hear about the juvenile diabetes, sensitivities to red wine and the asthma of her other cousins. He concluded that Kate did indeed have an auto-immune illness and even went so far as to guess that she was also a chronic fatigue (Epstein-Barr) patient, probably triggered by the mononucleosis she had when she was sixteen. Dr. Bihari wanted Kate to start on LDN immediately and after four weeks he wanted to have run some blood tests to see if the Epstein-Barr virus was still in her system.

Dr. Bihari hoped that Kate's energy levels would increase on LDN and that no additional medications would be needed, but should she not improve he mentioned an additional prescription that she might need. Kate was amazed that he was able to pinpoint some symptoms that she had forgotten to tell him about, particularly difficulty with short term memory and occasional flare ups of hives for no apparent reason. Kate felt that Dr. Bihari was one of the first doctors who ever listened to her.

Dr. Bihari also recommended that Rosemary take LDN as a preventative measure considering six out of nine siblings on her dad's side died of cancer. They left his office filled with hope. Kate started LDN Monday December 15th 2003. I was so happy for her and really hoped that she would live happily ever after. I still hope that Kate lives happily ever after.

Christmas 2003 was a wonderful Christmas, probably one of my best. Mom, Dad, Annie and Neilus came to visit us again and Neilus had a follow-up appointment with Dr. Bihari on December 17th. When I went to JFK airport to pick them up I immediately noticed how well Neilus looked. He looked great, but I couldn't put my finger on it as to why. His shake was still visible, but it had reduced since the previous year.

Neilus and I headed into New York on our own for the follow-up consultation. Dr. Bihari's secretary, Bill, greeted us when we came out of the elevator on that visit. Bill had family in Roscommon, in Ireland, he told us.

Dr. Bihari called us in and expressed sincere gratitude for my efforts in Ireland with regard to LDN and MS. He was receiving many phone calls from Ireland with reference to my name. He was very excited and told me that he was hopeful trials in Africa would start in February 2003 for HIV and AIDS.

Dr. Bihari also showed me a copy of a fax he received informing him that the question of an LDN trial for MS was recently raised in the Scottish Parliament. I asked him to make me a copy of that fax so I could investigate more. I told him that my wish was for a clinical trial in Ireland for

LDN and MS and explained that there were many people who were eager to help in Ireland, not because of me, but because LDN was working for MS.

I asked Dr. Bihari outright how far would he be willing to go to help get a trial get off the ground. I told him that my plan would be to get him on the airwaves first, then with the help of the media mount pressure on the Government to take initiative. He said that he would do all in his power to carry out a clinical trial with a reputable body. He told me that he wouldn't charge anything to set up a trial. All he would ask for is basic flight and board. The only thing the Government would have to pay for would be the actual trial which he would set up free of charge. He estimated the cost of a trial to be about two million Euro at the time.

I could see and clearly remember feeling that Dr. Bihari genuinely felt for all of the families that could be helped by LDN. He desperately wanted LDN to hit the masses in his lifetime. What also struck me, at the time, was his lack of desire for any personal gain. It did not seem to matter to him. I was humbled by his humility because he wanted nothing in return for the scientific recognition of LDN. I could not imagine how anybody could not like the guy.

Dr. Bihari proceeded with the consultation and examined Neilus. He concluded that not only did Neilus not decline, he had actually improved modestly. He said that Neilus' facial expression was much better and as soon as he said that I realized that was what I couldn't put my finger on at the airport. It was true, Neilus had more facial expression. Also, Dr. Bihari believed that Neilus' gait was swifter and his arms were less rigid.

Then Dr. Bihari shared with us that he had nine Parkinson's patients at that time on LDN and all were stable. Some had more improvements than others he stated. Overall he was delighted with Neilus' progress. Neilus and I were so happy. Once again we were filled with hope.

Before we left his office, Dr. Bihari convinced me to start taking LDN because of Mom's breast cancer. He explained that because she was struck post-menopause, the chances of me being at risk were reduced, but if I were his daughter he would prefer me on it. I told him that I was waiting for something to happen first, but he told me that he would not mess around. He said that breast cancer can be a dominant gene and that he wouldn't take any chances.

It was amazing how different my questions became once I was asked to take LDN myself. I told Dr. Bihari that my concern was that my body would become dependant on LDN for endorphin production and if ever I went off it I would plummet. He assured me that would never happen. He said that if I took LDN, my endorphins would be raised to their correct level and if I came off it they would just go back to pre LDN levels.

"Prevention is always best!" he said.

If my endorphins were low, Dr. Bihari told me that nothing, except LDN, would raise them sufficiently. He assured me that I would not be able to boost them enough naturally even if I spent all day everyday making love or eating chocolate. He told me that people already tried to get the LDN effect naturally and couldn't and advised me not to try to reinvent the wheel. If my endorphins were low, Dr. Bihari explained that whatever I was genetically predisposed to acquire would most likely appear within a couple of years. I had experienced sufficient stress in recent years to believe that my endorphins could have taken a hit and Mom's cancer and Neilus' Parkinson's convinced me that I was genetically vulnerable to get *something,* so I decided to start LDN. I have to admit that I would have been more comfortable with a blood-test that proved the state of my endorphins, but I started LDN anyway. I would also have liked the promise of a blood-test after a few months on LDN that would prove to me that my endorphin levels had actually improved, but as I said before, such a test is apparently not that straightforward. I think that such a blood test would greatly help. At least it would be one form of measurable evidence seeing as proof in improvements with MS is so elusive.

Chapter 23

"We all live with the objective of being happy;
our lives are all different and yet the same."

Anne Frank

My house had plenty of LDN so I popped one on December 17th before my prescription arrived. I woke at 2:00 a.m., completely alert and ready to start my day. I could not get back to sleep until about 4:00 a.m.. This lasted for about a week.

Since then I have noticed that my hair and nails grow faster, I sweat more and I need less sleep. The rapid hair growth and sweating are not the most endearing of feminine traits and are ones I would never want exaggerated or publicized, but they are manageable. I have also noticed that it is easier to track my fertility on LDN because it seems to exaggerate the signs. I should point out that Natural Family Planning is not something at which I have ever excelled, but

LDN did help me to recognize the signs more easily. Over-all, I feel good on LDN, but I have always been blessed with good health so I am not any example as to whether or not the drug is really effective. However, it is a good sign that I have been taking LDN for five years and am still alive and as healthy as ever. Whether or not it has done me any good, I don't know, but I do know that it has not done me any harm. Noel will yell at me for the next over-share, but I do notice that I have developed a couple of facial whiskers. Tia assured me that all women my age get whiskers and that it is perfectly normal and easily managed, so maybe the whiskers are independent of LDN. The only thing I know for sure is that Tia thinks everything is normal.

Kate, Rosemary and I started LDN around the same time that Christmas in 2003. We exchanged e-mail daily to report on our progress and I enjoyed getting to know them. Rosemary had no problems adjusting whatsoever. She never noticed a thing, not even a sleepless night. Kate, like me, had difficulty sleeping initially. We were wired for about a week and swore that we looked like we got hit by a bus. It was fun though, because we were in it together and I was confident that it would pass because I had been track-ing LDN for some time. Kate and I adjusted, and started to sleep normally, but her energy levels did not come back. I felt dreadful about that. I felt that I probably raised her hopes too high with my optimism.

I could not understand why she did not seem to be re-sponding to LDN and I found it difficult to accept. Then, thank God, Kate announced that she was pregnant. She and her family were ecstatic. It was wonderful news. At the time, Dr. Bihari advised his patients to come off LDN for pregnancy, although he had some patients with AIDS who remained on it for the duration and had healthy babies. Un-til the drug is clinically proven he recommended to play it safe. Kate stopped taking LDN towards the end of January 2004 and gave birth to a beautiful baby boy, Matthew, on October 14th. She was Dr. Bihari's first Samters patient, but not on the drug long enough to prove or disprove its effectiveness for Samters. Kate intended to resume LDN after she finished breastfeeding Matthew. Then Luke arrived. And then came Brynn. Thank God, Kate had three remarkably healthy pregnancies. She is delighted with motherhood, a complete natural by all accounts, and her excitement is quite contagious. I hope that should she ever need to resume LDN in the future, it will work for her.

I mentioned earlier that since 2002, my brother, Dr. Phil Boyle, has used LDN in his practice as part of his protocol to help some of his patients conceive. Initially, he kept some patients on LDN for the first trimester of their pregnancy to make sure that the pregnancy was strong enough to sustain itself without LDN. Phil was reluctant to take his patients off LDN until he was certain that the pregnancy was strong enough to survive. Remarkably, he even has some patients who chose to stay on LDN for their entire pregnancy because they believed it best for both the mother and child. Phil monitors all of his patients very closely and would have insisted they stopped LDN at any point if there was any reason for concern. He also knew that pregnant women in the U.S. have taken up to 100 mg of Naltrexone daily for drug addiction, for the entire duration of pregnancy without ill-effect to them or their babies. To think that people have successfully taken LDN, at such a high dose, for the duration of a pregnancy speaks volumes for the safety of the drug.

I should also point out that most women do not need LDN when they are pregnant. The decision to stay on LDN when pregnant would have to highly depend on why a person is taking LDN in the first place. If LDN is being used to treat a very serious condition, then it would make little sense to stop taking it when pregnant. Would I stay on LDN if I was pregnant? To be honest, I wouldn't unless I absolutely had to. If I had HIV, cancer, MS or an aggressive autoimmune disease I would. If I had a less serious condition, I wouldn't, but I would resume LDN as soon as the baby was born or sooner if the pregnancy triggered a major relapse. I know that people who have taken LDN for an entire pregnancy have pushed back the frontiers and removed a lot of the fear, but not all of it. And besides, these are difficult questions that I can't really answer. To imagine a situation is very different to the reality of one. The decision to take LDN when pregnant would have to be a personal one based on an individual's circumstance, history and comfort zone. But, without doubt, pregnancy is another major reason why the drug needs a large scale clinical trial. However, for now, it is nice to know that LDN need not be totally ruled out during pregnancy.

What is remarkable about LDN is the wide range of diseases it helps. It links so many diseases of the immune system together. A trial would shed some much needed light on how the immune system actually works. I firmly believe that LDN could greatly complement and boost many other therapies, including stem cells. It is very likely that LDN would make many promising treatments even better. It would have to because it boosts the immune system. The more I think about it, a large scale LDN trial is simply imperative because it holds far too much promise to ignore.

After we celebrated Christmas and rang in 2004, Mom, Dad, Annie and Neilus flew back to Ireland. I decided to follow-up with Pat Kenny and investigate what was going on with the Scottish Parliament. There seemed to be so much happening and it was exciting.

166

Rosemary shared my interest. She used the internet to keep up to date with what people were saying about LDN. I loved conversing with her and e-mailed her regularly. It amazed me how easily I could open up to her on all levels. She said that she enjoyed our connection and looked forward to hearing from me, so a friendship developed that I will always cherish.

I learned to channel my enthusiasm for writing to Rosemary into this story, which will hopefully entice people to investigate LDN, either for themselves or a loved one and keep the snowball rolling. This book that you are reading is in fact based on a collection of e-mails I sent to Rosemary because I wanted her to understand everything. I am grateful that she tapped into a skill I never knew I possessed because I desperately wanted to share this story. I wish everyone would meet a Rosemary.

I would love if this book would grant me some celebrity status that I could use along with my newfound wealth to actually privately fund an LDN trial. That may seem difficult and sound a touch overly optimistic, but believe me, it might be easier than attracting the attention of current celebrities. I never realized how difficult it actually is to get the attention of a celebrity. How many crazies can there possibly be out there bothering them all on a daily basis?

I started with Pat Kenny, a popular TV broadcaster in Ireland. The story seemed right up his alley. I thought that he would even thank me for bringing it to his attention. I sent him a follow-up letter in January 2004, 2005, 2006 and 2007, but he didn't respond. I still can't believe that despite my persistence, he managed to ignore me.

I have nothing at all against Pat Kenny or any celebrity whom I tried to entice. I cannot blame anyone with power to influence and personal credibility to maintain for treating the matter somewhat dubiously. It requires someone, somewhere, with position and power, to take a leap of faith. But, as more time passes, the required leap keeps getting smaller and smaller, as the anecdotal testimonies multiply and preliminary small scale trials complete. Pat Kenny will run some sort of a story on LDN someday.

The initial letter that I wrote to him in September 2003, did serve much purpose though. I also sent the letter to my list of MS contacts in Ireland, and e-mailed it to friends and family all over the world. It was probably the first insight many had in to our lives with MS and it touched some people deeply. Everyone wanted to do something to help. Noel's Dad called me to ask if he could give the letter to the doctors he knew in Donegal. Friends whom I hadn't really talked to in years printed out copies and literally distributed them to strangers on the street. I laughed one day when I logged on to the internet because a guy I never met from Letterkenny got my e-mail address from the MS society in Letterkenny in Ireland, and sent me a copy of the letter and inquired if I knew anything about it. I really felt as if word was getting out. The LDN website editor, Dr. Gluck, also e-mailed me to ask me if he could use the letter on the official LDN website. I agreed.

I should have told Noel that his story was on the internet, but I didn't and a funny thing happened. Noel was thriving on LDN. As always he was high on life, but his latest kick was a serious urge to give back to the community. He decided to participate in the organization of a Christian retreat called Cornerstone that he attended the previous year. His role was a witness speaker whereby he had to give an account as to how God helped him in life. He thought that it would be a good thing to share his epiphany with people. During the retreat he got to know many people, one of whom told him that he read Noel's story on the internet because his sister had MS. Of course, I knew this man's wife and gave her all of the information and asked her to pass it on to her sister-in-law. Noel came home and knew that it could only have been me who posted his MS story on the internet. He asked me about it and I confessed. Thankfully, the glow of Cornerstone saved me.

I often think of that witness speech Noel gave. He let me read it and it hit me deeply that it would be a much nicer world if everybody had a little more "Noel" in them. The speech told about his childhood in Belfast, his lonely experiences at boarding school and his depression in London. Then, it gave a brief and humble description of his epiphany and continued to describe his MS diagnosis and progression. I think that it sounded like a pretty depressing existence to any normal person, but I couldn't believe the last line. He actually felt that he had to tell the guys that his life wasn't perfect! He even qualified that statement by sharing with them that he "still fights with his wife over stupid stuff." That was pretty inspiring.

Chapter 24

*"Whatever you vividly imagine, ardently desire,
sincerely believe, and enthusiastically act upon,
must inevitably come to pass!"*

Paul J. Meyer

I t was early 2004 when I came across an article in *New
Horizon's* Winter 2003 issue, by the Brewer Science
Library in Wisconsin. It was written by Christina White
and titled "LDN Results for Multiple Sclerosis Patients."
She stated that she first wrote about some of the dramatic
results that Dr. Bihari had reported with LDN use five
years previously. Her first article on LDN was entitled
"Only One Pill A Day Keeps Some Cancers At Bay" and it
was published in *New Horizon's* Spring 1999 issue. Since
then, this was her fifth article following up on LDN and
very detailed. It included a reference to the Goodshape
website and said that it was one of the first websites to post

LDN information. Christina wrote that Goodshape heard about LDN from one of their subscribers who posted on his site and she said that Goodshape called her to discuss results with it for various diseases. She commented on how the word was spreading like wildfire through the web based MS Community and she printed many LDN testimonies and clarified that all of the results were anecdotal. It was a well written account and it felt good to see LDN in print again. There have been hundreds of LDN articles published since then, but not enough because there are still millions of people out there who need to hear about LDN yesterday, but haven't.

Shortly after reading Christina's article I decided to investigate what was going on in Scotland. I read the information Dr. Bihari copied for me in December. It stated that on Friday 12th December 2003, LDN was formally addressed in the Scottish Parliament. That sounded very promising. I knew that a trial in Scotland would do just as good as one in Ireland.

A woman named Irene Oldfather asked the Scottish Executive what information it had regarding LDN in the treatment of MS and of current prescribing practices for LDN in Ireland and North America. She asked them to compare the cost of current therapies with the cost of LDN. She also directly asked whether they would consider funding clinical trials to monitor the effectiveness of LDN in the treatment of MS. That was what held my focus.

I posted on the Yahoo LDN message board to find out who was responsible for this. A couple named Lorna and Terry McDevitt, from Scotland, replied to me in private. Lorna was in her mid-forties and she started LDN to treat her MS in April 2003. She was so impressed with the results that she and her husband were trying as best they could to get the drug into a clinical trial in Scotland.

The first thing Lorna noticed on LDN was that the numbness in her back improved. Then her stiffness and fatigue began to fade. One morning she got up, worked on her computer, cooked and tidied up and was absolutely delighted with herself, because prior to taking LDN she could not do anything before late morning. Lorna and Terry told me that they would update me as soon as they got word from the Scottish Parliament and I promised them that I would keep them informed of events in Ireland.

On January 13th 2004 the Scottish Parliament replied to the questions. Basically they said that they had no information on LDN and MS. They said that they were not directly funding any research, including clinical trials on MS. That was mainly due to the fact that no research proposals on MS had been received in recent years they claimed. They stated that they would be pleased to consider research proposals for innovative MS studies of a sufficiently high standard. They also added that these proposals would be subject to the usual peer and committee review. At least the Scottish Parliament was now aware of LDN I thought. It took time to send them a formal proposal and once received, it was finally rejected. I don't even think it was debated.

Meanwhile in Galway, Robert and others were organizing an LDN conference in The Menlo Park Hotel for January 16th 2003 at 8:00 p.m.. The event was advertised in the Galway MS Newsletter and broadcast on local radio. I informed Lorna and Terry, and they flew over at the last minute to attend. The audience spilled over from the conference room out into the hall and Robert spoke to the crowd about LDN. Many people I know attended and by all accounts he gave a remarkable account backed by his wife, Alma. Lorna also told her story and I was told that she was a major asset to the event. After that conference more people got my e-mail from the Galway MS Society and the word continued to spread.

At this stage, a pharmacist in Gort, County Galway, named Brendan Quinn, started to supply LDN in Ireland and was starting to become inundated with queries. Unfortunately, Brendan also had a loved one who was diagnosed with MS. He read everything on the internet about LDN and thoroughly investigated. Also, Robert managed to persuade his neurologist in Galway to prescribe his LDN and the Western Health Board agreed to pay for it under the Long Term Illness Act and Brendan agreed to make it for him. The snowball continued to roll.

After much research, Brendan started to prepare LDN for many people wanting to try it. For some he was making it up in liquid form and for others he was importing the capsules from Martindale Pharmaceuticals in the UK. He could see positive results, but he could not explain them. We started to converse regularly and the more we talked, the more driven we became for a proper clinical scientific trial. The reports that I got back from people starting LDN kept me focused. It was worth every effort. The last time I spoke with Quinn's Pharmacy, they had acquired the technology to make LDN capsules onsite and had over 500 patients on LDN.

It is important to point out that not everybody wanted to try LDN. There was then and still is now, a personal risk people feel that they have to take in order to try it. There always will be that feeling for some people, until a large scale clinical trial is carried out. It is important to realize that there were plenty of people whom I could not convince to try it. Like I said before, as long as they had heard about LDN, my job was done.

Chapter 25

"Where does one go from a world of insanity?
Somewhere on the other side of despair."

T.S. Eliot

There are many people with whom I love to keep in touch in Ireland and I make a point of getting together with them every time I go home for a visit. One of these people is Maire Thornton. She was my hockey coach when I was in school and because we traveled so much together, we got to know each other very well and became good friends. I was always aware that her sister had MS. Shortly after Noel started LDN, I gave Maire all of the information on LDN and she passed it on, but her sister opted for chemotherapy instead. She was afraid of LDN. She wanted her neurologist to tell her to take LDN. Although the LDN campaign has come a long, long way, we are still years from that milestone.

Then Maire developed a neurological problem that confused all of her doctors. She had a few uncomfortable years and was considering trying LDN herself to see if it would help her. Given the fact that her sister had MS and her own doctors were confused, Maire wanted to try LDN just to see if it would offer her any relief, but she lacked the energy to get the prescription. It is still not an easy task to get an LDN prescription in Ireland. Unfortunately, I know for a fact that there are many Maires in Ireland.

Actually I am pretty sure that there are many Maires worldwide. People who have educated themselves on LDN and clearly see that it is safer than aspirin, will not break the bank and has so much anecdotal evidence that they are desperate to try it, but just can't. Many doctors are not willing to write a prescription for LDN and if they do they don't want it known. That is a crazy situation, but also a reality. I want to remove the fear.

Patients in the U.S. have had to sign waivers stating that they will not hold the doctor responsible for whatever happens to them on LDN in order to get it prescribed. Some people have actually pretended to have a drug or alcohol problem in order to get a naltrexone prescription. Then they crush the naltrexone and add water themselves in order to home brew a lumpy nightly shot. But many people give up because they don't have the energy to fight the system or the confidence to home brew.

Thankfully, there are a handful of doctors who went to the trouble of investigating the drug and deduced that LDN is a safe prescription to write and are not afraid. If more doctors would investigate, more fear would be removed, but until there is a large scale clinical trial there will be a reluctance on the part of many doctors to seriously consider the benefits of LDN. That makes for an incredibly frustrating situation for too many people. Any doctor willing to investigate the drug should have no trouble writing a script. There is more than enough documented evidence of its safety and efficacy. There is absolutely nothing to be afraid of.

Etta Apgar, is another friend of mine from the Moms Group at Nativity. Her Dad was a cop in Florida for most of his life. He retired, and for years they suspected that he had Lyme Disease. Then, in his mid-fifties he was diagnosed with MS and told that there was no treatment for him. His neurologist told him that he was too old for any of the MS therapies. Also, it sounded as though he had progressive MS because it was progressing rapidly. Etta has shared many horrific stories about her dad's near death experiences as a result of his MS, such as falling head first through glass doors. She is deeply concerned for him, but cannot get him a prescription for LDN because his doctor has never heard about it and that is good enough for her dad. Like many, he wants to do what his doctor thinks is best for him. This drives his daughter insane. That is a very tough situation, but I can understand her dad. It is by no means unreasonable to want to listen to your lifelong doctor.

Then there is Ava Crawford from Pennsylvania. She is my friend Rachel's husband's aunt. Noel and I visited Rachel and her husband, Mike, in October 2003, shortly after they moved to Ohio. I made a point of meeting Ava who was visiting her sister in Ohio, at the time, because Mike told me that Ava had MS. Ava was about fifty and blind. The distance she could walk was limited, but mentally she was very alert.

There are fighters and then there is Ava. She did not have an easy life, but she certainly made the most of it and I believe that she inspires everyone she meets. She certainly inspires me. Ava took all of the LDN information I had and thoroughly investigated it. She followed up on everything

and e-mailed me with many queries and concerns. She took
the information to her neurologist and literally insisted on a
prescription. She had a good relationship with her neurologist and he respected her judgment. She was on Avonex at
the time and made the personal decision, which is never
easy, to come off it. That made her neurologist very nervous, but it didn't bother Ava once she made up her mind.
LDN was not compounded in Pennsylvania so I taught her
how to home brew. Five years later, Ava told me that her
neurologist still wants her to go back on Avonex or to start
Copaxone, but she refuses because her quality of life since
she quit Avonex and went on LDN is so much better. Also,
her MRIs since starting LDN have not shown any new le-
sions. She feels that LDN is working for her. Ava is glad
that she discovered LDN. I think that everyone with an
autoimmune disease who has discovered LDN is glad that
they did. It is worth fighting for.

By February 2004, I had no doubt that Dr. Bihari had
discovered something with the potential to help millions,
but I still didn't see the whole picture clearly. I was so focused on MS it was as if I had tunnel vision. My main focus was Ireland because the few MS Societies I contacted
in the U.S. totally ignored me. They didn't want to hear
about LDN, so I basically gave up on spreading the word in
the U.S.. I desperately wanted them to take the matter seriously, but I was hit with a prewritten response every time.
My dealings with the National Multiple Sclerosis Society
(NMSS) in the U.S. have been very discouraging, to say the
least, and I have stopped donating money to them. Cold and
corporate is the only way I can describe them. Instead of
them actively investigating what can only be described as
overwhelming anecdotal evidence as to the effectiveness of
LDN for MS, they stuck their head in the sand and said that
they cannot comment or help in any shape or form until the

drug is clinically proven. Surely it is the duty of the MS Societies to help the fast growing web based MS community set the LDN record straight? If not, it should be. Maybe their name needs to be adjusted also in order to clarify their primary interests.

Many years have passed since my first dealings with the NMSS and my feelings have changed very little. After a huge amount of pressure from grassroots movements, they gave Penn State 44,000 U.S. dollars for LDN research, but it is not enough. It is nowhere near enough and they know that. Now and then they mention LDN, but they need to do a great deal more. It is unacceptable that the NMSS continue to shamelessly push expensive, toxic medicines (that don't work) on people with MS when they know that LDN is not only safer and cost-effective, but working a heck of a lot better for most people. I would love to pull their head from the sand.

Sometimes, the enormity of the battle for a trial would get me down. It can feel very frustrating and depressing to think that the battle is such an uphill struggle because of the lack of financial profit LDN holds. That is so fundamentally wrong. It highlights something so wrong with the way in which the world works that it makes my blood boil. Nobody should ever profit from sick people. Period. Billion dollar industries based on maintaining diseases should be illegal.

I learned that maintaining illness is more profitable than curing it. I learned that sick people make others very rich and I don't like that. I also learned that I am too small to change any of it. For now, things just are. I would bet my life though, that LDN therapy is not the first, nor will it be the last, effective therapy to be blocked by corporate giants. When I say blocked, I really mean ignored because that is all they have to do. Pharmaceutical companies worldwide, should never have been allowed to become as powerful as they have. And yet, I appreciate the fact that the same giants protect us from gimmicks and quackery, but the balance is blatantly wrong. There is no balance and that is a big problem. And here is the kicker: the bad guy is actually invisible. There is nobody I can call to yell at even. I can't point to any corporate giant and say they go out of their way to actively prevent LDN from reaching the masses. People who do that come across as crazy. If a company decides not to investigate LDN, then they are hardly bad guys. They are, in fact, very smart businessmen. The problem lies within the fabric of our entire health system. The whole system needs to be dismantled and redefined. A job much too big for me.

I gave up on the U.S. because I could not see a large scale LDN trial enticing any pharmaceutical company to investigate and my focus became Ireland, only because they stood to make money on the outcome of a successful trial.

I shared my frustration with Rosemary who knew what I was trying to achieve and for some reason understood me very well. She always kept our conversations light and I enjoyed her gentle wisdom. There were times I know that I really needed it. Amazingly, Rosemary never agreed or disagreed with my perceptions, but she always listened. She was always there for me. I couldn't ask for a wiser mentor or better friend.

One day Rosemary told me that she thought that I needed a wider audience. She had seen an Oprah Special Report that Christmas about AIDS in Africa and remembered that Dr. Bihari was looking at doing a trial in South Africa for LDN and AIDS. Rosemary deduced that Oprah would be interested to hear about an LDN trial in South Africa, and that if Oprah became convinced of LDN's potential then she would most likely do everything she could to help LDN reach the masses. I decided to investigate.

Chapter 26

"Most of the important things in the world have been accomplished by people who have kept on trying when there seemed to be no hope at all."

Dale Carnegie

I don't watch TV very much so I was not too familiar with Oprah. I knew very little about her, but the more I read, the more I liked her and the more I understood what Rosemary was saying. It was clear that if I could convince Oprah of the potential LDN held for AIDS in South Africa, she would do all in her power to get LDN to the people. That would have to involve a scientific clinical trial, and if a clinical trial proved effective for AIDS and HIV by boosting the immune system, then I figured that the MS community leaders would have to sit up and take notice.

Oprah recorded a remarkable documentary on AIDS in South Africa and it was aired during Christmas 2003. I imagine that she made her point with millions, me included. It was a human approach where she met and befriended real people dying of AIDS, leaving behind real children. Her main focus was the on the children and I think that anybody who saw the reality of the lives some people in South Africa live, would have to think twice before ever complaining again.

The show was called Christmas Kindness and it took Oprah a year to make it. She hired one hundred people to get the word out that the children were invited to a Christmas party, and she brought along many gifts. She even referred to it as the single greatest experience of her life.

Oprah gave each child a pair of shoes and a photo of themselves. Each girl received a black doll, and each boy, a football and she also gave away jeans. She made Christmas special for tens of thousands of children from the most wretched of villages far too familiar with death.

From an interview Oprah did with Diane Sawyer, I learned that every minute in South Africa, sixty-four people die of AIDS. They have left behind a whole generation of children without parents, food or any way out.

There may be as many as eleven million of these orphans, according to the United Nations. It's as if every child under the age of nineteen in New York were left to raise themselves. It is absolutely tragic.

South Africa's president, at the time, Thabo Mbeki, had long described poverty as the biggest threat and killer in South Africa and had expressed doubts, both about the link between HIV and AIDS and the extent to which the disease had spread in South Africa. But the South African government later approved the provision of AIDS drugs to HIV positive people through the public health system. That was a significant step forward, but they need more. They need LDN.

Educating myself on the enormity of the AIDS epidemic was a personal growth experience for me. It hit me on a level I didn't know I could reach. The real potential promise LDN held, according to Dr. Bihari, slowly sunk in. It went so far beyond MS, that MS actually seemed small in the grand scheme of things. I remembered everything Dr. Bihari told me about AIDS and HIV from when I first phoned him. I remembered him mentioning during my last visit with him in December, that he was very excited and eagerly anticipating a trial in South Africa for LDN and AIDS. I had no doubt that Oprah would indeed be very interested.

At this point, I wanted Oprah to know about LDN regardless of whether the MS community leaders took notice or not. I also had no doubt that Dr. Bihari was right. I felt no reason to doubt him because what he was saying about MS and Parkinson's seemed to be holding true. If what he said proved to be true for AIDS and HIV, the implications were staggering. I began to get excited about the prospect of a trial. Dr. Bihari's claims are difficult to believe, but it comes down to one question in my mind. What if he is right? What if even half of what he says proves to be true? I am certain that he is partly right because I have seen what LDN can do, so the question has to be: How right is he?

Dr. Bihari claims that 4.5 mg LDN actually prevents HIV developing into full blown AIDS if the patient's CD4 count is greater than 300. How unbelievable is that? I already mentioned that his early work consisted of helping those afflicted with drug and alcohol abuse and that his work extended to the HIV and AIDS community in the 80's. He published a paper in 1986 that was presented in 1988 to the International AIDS Conference in Stockholm, Sweden. His paper described in detail a placebo controlled LDN HIV/AIDS clinical study. In 2003, Dr. Bihari was monitoring twenty patients with HIV who had refused anti-viral drugs for many years, and continued to remain healthy on LDN alone. Also, 90% of his patients with AIDS who were treated with LDN in conjunction with antiretroviral therapy showed no detectable level of the virus after eight years. This is a substantially higher success rate than for any reported AIDS treatment group.

I cannot deny that it sounds too good to be true, but it gets even better. With local manufacture in South Africa, LDN would cost no more than 10 U.S. dollars per patient per year. And finally, without wanting to sound like an LDN commercial, but because LDN is a simple pill taken nightly, if clinically proven, it would hold great advantages over the combination antiviral regiments. Namely, it can be taken with discretion, which is a huge plus given the cultural stigma that accompanies AIDS and HIV victims, and it has no side-effects or need for medical supervision. These are life saving advantages for South Africa. It certainly sounds like a wonder drug, but by all accounts it is a wonder drug worth investigating because the promise it holds is phenomenal. I cannot help but constantly wonder exactly how right is Dr. Bihari?

Once I had the picture clear in my mind I set out to write Oprah a letter. Before I did that I read her biography to try to figure her out. It is only as I write this story do I realize that I have a unique way of approaching situations. I quickly deduced that she must be bombarded with mail so Rosemary suggested I call Dr. Bihari to ask him if he could give me anything to make my letter stand out.

Dr. Bihari had seen Oprah's Christmas Special and thought at the time that it would be wonderful if she knew about LDN. He told me that he had a great deal of respect for Oprah and all the work she was doing in South Africa. He was very appreciative of my efforts and delighted that

Rosemary prompted me. He remembered Rosemary from Kate's Samters consultation in December. Dr. Bihari warned me that he had tried to contact various celebrities in the past and concluded that it was by no means an easy task.

I asked him if he would tell me about the upcoming trial. He told me that there was a strong possibility that a trial was going to happen in Mali in February 2004 for LDN and AIDS and HIV. He was so excited that I could hear it in his voice.

The interest was sparked by a twenty-four-year-old from Mali who was studying to get his MBA in Chicago and became familiar with Dr. Bihari's work. His father was a man of position in the Islamic National Bank in Saudi Arabia, and good friends with the President of Mali. Dr. Bihari was told by the young man's father that the President had agreed to let him fly over and meet the planning commission to set up a trial. He was anxiously awaiting a letter from the President of Mali to confirm this. Dr. Bihari planned to get his visa and head over there as soon as the letter arrived.

I asked him what he thought would be the best way for me to approach Oprah. I asked should I wait until he got back and wondered if he would keep a journal or take pictures that I could use. He said that all I needed to get her attention in his opinion would be a copy of the letter he was waiting to receive from the President. He figured that would be enough to get her attention. He said that he would contact me as soon as the letter arrived and fax me a copy. I was very excited when I hung up the phone and could not wait to share his positive response with Rosemary. She thought that it was wonderful that Dr. Bihari was on board and agreed that the situation was exciting. Immediately, I set to work on the letter for Oprah.

The letter basically asked Oprah to take a leap of faith in Dr. Bihari. The letter gave a history of Dr. Bihari and went on to detail the promise LDN held for AIDS and HIV based on the 1986 placebo trial and his patients at the time. It told of the Developing Nations Project Dr. Bihari initiated to reach out to the developing world and ended with my family MS, Parkinson's and Breast Cancer stories with reference to my perception of Dr. Bihari's humble and compassionate character. I sent a copy of the letter to Dr. Bihari to make sure it was medically correct and asked him if the letter had arrived from the President of Mali. The letter had not arrived. Since then, I have learned that things take a great deal longer than I would like.

In February 2004, I decided to send my letter to Oprah on its own. I asked her to bridge the gap between Dr. Bihari and South Africa. I intended to follow up with the letter from Mali. I have to say, whatever about Pat Kenny ignoring me, I outdid myself in trying to capture Oprah's attention.

Before I mailed the letter, I sent it to a list of family and friends, all of whom contributed something. It was Valentines so I decided to wait for a couple of days until after the mail rush. I imagined that a lot of crazies send Oprah Valentines Day cards. I scanned in a family picture at the end of the letter to make it more personal, I added my e-mail address, wrote a cover letter and used apple green paper. To be sad enough to know that apple green happens to be Oprah's favorite color is one thing, but to be so obvious about it is another. I now think that I probably scared the woman.

I would have scared her a great deal more if Rosemary didn't intervene. I was going to send Oprah fifty copies of the same letter because she had just turned fifty. I hoped to hit a cross section of her staff in the hope that one would find it worth passing on. I imagined a room full of people going through her sacks of mail and wanted fifty of them to read it. Rosemary put a halt to that crazy idea by suggesting that I test the system first instead of presuming it was at fault. She wanted me to give Oprah the benefit of the doubt initially, which sounded reasonable, so I did. Tia feared that fifty letters would prompt a visit from the FBI for stalking and joked that even bad publicity was better than none.

I turned a simple letter into "Operation Oprah" and there was huge relief when I finally sent it. I mailed it direct to Harpo. Of course I didn't just mail it, I sent it express, priority, delivery receipt written confirmation and certified. The young man at the post office looked at me that day and said "Gee Lady, you must want tickets for that show real bad." I laughed and said yes. I was very happy with the letter.

About a week or so later I received the written confirmation in my mailbox and noticed that the letter was received by a lady named Ana. I called Harpo Inc. in Chicago and asked to speak with her. She told me that she receives all of Oprah's mail and sorts it. It is then reviewed by the next level of people and whatever they find interesting goes to the research team and if the content passes research then it is brought direct to Oprah's attention.

Ana told me that fifty letters would have annoyed her intensely. I asked her what would be the best way to try to get Oprah's attention. She told me to watch a show and to note the names at the end and mail the names direct.

The names don't appear in New Jersey so I called my cousin, Sheila, in Chicago. She told me that her husband went on the Oprah show with his construction company, Liffey Construction, a while back when Oprah was doing a show on how to build panic rooms. It turned out that Sheila had a list of Oprah's entire senior staff, so I sent them all a copy of the letter and followed up with a phone call. I ended up dealing directly with a lady called Layla in Harpo. Layla assured me that they have received the entire story and it is in review. I am sure that Layla will call me any day now.

Chapter 27

*"Many people have a wrong idea of what constitutes
true happiness. It is not attained through self-gratification,
but through fidelity to a worthy purpose."*

Helen Keller

"Operation Oprah" developed into "Operation LDN." The AIDS angle completely consumed me for the next while. I thoroughly researched the South African Government. I read a great deal about Thabo Mbeki and wrote a letter to him. The letter was basically the same as the one I sent to Oprah except it lacked any emotional pleas. It was more of a business letter propositioning his Government to look into Dr. Bihari's work because it seemed to hold enormous potential for their Country. I also sent the letter to a cross section of the South African Government in the hope that one of them would take heed. As well as sending the letters in the mail

I also e-mailed them. Once again, as I write, it is obvious that the whole thing consumed me.

I was delighted and shocked to receive a prompt e-mail response from the South African Government. It was from Charmaine Fredericks and dated March 23rd 2004. It read:

Dear Ms Bradley

We hereby wish to acknowledge with thanks receipt of the correspondence for the Deputy President regarding the work of Dr. Bernard Bihari.

This has been forwarded to the Deputy President's Special Adviser, Mr. Siyabonga Mcetywa who will liaise with you in due course.

For your information, Mr. Mcetywa's contact details are: Tel.: +27 12 300 5310 Fax +27 12 323 3114

Yours sincerely
Administrative Secretary

That was exciting. I called the number in the letter and spoke with Mr. Mcetywa's secretary, Doreen, for about half an hour. She seemed very interested and assured me that she would pass on the information. I also received written confirmation in the mail dated May 13th from the Trade and Industry Ministry acknowledging receipt of the information with gratitude. That was also exciting. It is not everyday I get mail from a Government. I was delighted that at least they had the information. That was, however, the last I heard from South Africa.

I forwarded all correspondence to Oprah and her staff in the hope that she would take action, but I am still waiting. I learned that it is not easy to interest a celebrity, any celebrity.

I developed the "more the merrier" approach. I decided to tell as many celebrities as possible about LDN, focusing on those who publicize that they care about the AIDS epidemic. My compulsion was contagious and my friend, Coirle, in Ireland, joined my efforts and starting pumping out letters herself. She also kept LDN information which she downloaded from the internet in her car so that when she was driving around Galway she always had a printout available for people she believed would have interest.

Also, here in New Jersey, the Moms Group dispensed LDN information at every given opportunity. One day, a friend of mine called me on her cell phone from a pet store in New Jersey after she discovered that the owner had MS. It was a crazy thing for my friend to do and I laughed afterwards, but she did put me in touch with the lady who was very grateful and most interested in the information. I was delighted. It felt wonderful to have so much support from friends and family.

I wrote to Bono, Mary Robinson, Bishop Tutu and Nelson Mandela in the hope that someone would eventually have their curiosity piqued and carry the torch. It seemed almost incomprehensible to think that no one would take the time to check it out, but nobody replied.

On March 31st 2004, I wrote to the Bill and Melinda Gates Foundation. Rosemary noticed an article in the local paper that stated he had an online application form for research grants to help the AIDS Crisis. I found the application form and it seemed perfect for LDN. It was perfect because it was brief and straight to the point. I called Dr. Bihari to inform him and again he thought it worthwhile. I asked him how much I should request. His reply once again amazed me. He said that all that he would need to get an LDN trial in South Africa underway was 250,000 U.S. Dollars. I applied for the grant, but was declined. I respected how prompt they were in their reply. On April 1st 2004 I received a letter of rejection from Bill and Melinda. Part of it read:

"We agree that the work you describe will help to improve health in the developing world. However, it has been determined that the proposed activities are not among the current priorities for support by the Bill & Melinda Gates Foundation as our focus is on HIV prevention rather than treatment at this time. In order to stay focused on our highest priorities, we must unfortunately decline funding for many worthwhile projects."

It is funny, but when you really look at it, the world isn't that big and I was quickly running out of options. On the MS front, I e-mailed Meredith Viera after a couple of friends prompted me to. They read her husband's story in the local paper. I also fired off the same letter to Montel Williams, but once again nobody replied.

On the Parkinson's front I tried Michael J Fox, but he didn't answer. I finally concluded that writing to celebrities, although worth a shot, was futile.

In September 2007, after years of preparatory efforts by many LDN advocates and without the help of any celebrity, the Institutional Review Board in Bamako, the capital of Mali, finally approved plans for a clinical trial of LDN in people who are HIV-infected—the first scientific study of LDN for HIV/AIDS in Africa. Dr. Jaquelyn McCandless assumed the responsibilities of "Expatriate Clinical Monitor" for the medical aspects of the trial.

It is January 2009 now, and the study is not finished. It is taking much longer than anticipated because of the huge stigma (especially for women) that causes people to fear getting tested until it is too late for them to be in the study, which is more about preventing HIV developing into AIDS, rather than the treatment of AIDS. The study involves three study groups: LDN treatment only; LDN plus antiretroviral drugs; and only antiretroviral drugs. The volunteer subjects must be eighteen years of age or older and must have reduced CD4 counts in the 275 to 475 cells range at the outset. Laboratory studies are rechecked at twelve-week intervals.

The research team is led by Dr. Abdel Kader Traore and other health officials at the University Hospital in Bamako. Irmat Pharmacy of Manhattan volunteered to supply all of the LDN required and matching placebo capsules at no cost. In addition, the study includes counseling aimed at improving preventive health practices for women and children. The latest information on that LDN trial and all other LDN trials can be found on the not for profit, official LDN website: www.ldninfo.org.

Chapter 28

"In all things it is better to hope than to despair."
Johann Wolfgang von Goethe

In April 2004, I asked Noel if he would like to take a trip back to Ireland, but he couldn't because he was very busy at work. He told me to make the trip with the children during their school break, so I booked our flights to Ireland for April 23rd 2004, for nine days.

On April 18th, my friend, Paula, organized a team from the Moms Group to do an MS Walk in Ridgewood to raise funds for the NMSS. I was reluctant to participate, but I wanted to show my personal support for Paula (who was thriving on LDN) so I went along. The weather was beautiful and we all gathered at Graydon Pool in Ridgewood, New Jersey.

I could not contain myself when I saw all of the different teams and all of the people directly affected by MS. I wrote out the LDN website address along with my name, address, phone number and e-mail on fifty pieces of paper and ran to each team and distributed the information to the members. I explained the theory to most. I was delighted to have the support of good friends from the Moms Group for the walk. I wasn't sure if I was brave enough to approach complete strangers, but my friends kept the pep talks running, pinpointed the targets and made it happen. I am still in touch with five people from that day who have MS. All five went on LDN around that time and continue to thrive today.

There was so much happening regarding MS and LDN on the internet at that time and it was very exciting. Many people were putting in tremendous personal effort to get the word out and help others. There were so many people reaching out and sharing personal, but wonderful stories and experiences. The MS community really had momentum.

A lady named Edwina from Cork, joined forces with Robert in Galway, Lorna and Terrence in Scotland and another lady named Linda in England. They put together an internet petition asking for a clinical trial of LDN and MS for people to sign. To date the petition has 10,488 signatures. When enough are gathered it will be presented to the Irish Government and others. That is another item worth googling.

Edwina is in her mid twenties and has Relapsing Remitting MS. I remember her from the summer of 2003 because I e-mailed her about LDN along with everyone else who had their details on the MS Ireland website. She investigated LDN, and when she decided to try it, she had great difficulty getting her prescription. She ended up getting it from Dr. Lawrence in Wales, but had to wait quite a while for an appointment. Thank God, like Robert, she went on

LDN and in turn has helped and educated numerous others. Fatigue and bladder control were the main improvements experienced almost immediately by Edwina.

As with Rosemary's daughter Kate, Edwina also conceived shortly after she started LDN. She was on LDN for six weeks when she discovered she was pregnant and like Kate, she decided to stop LDN because she didn't feel comfortable taking any medication during pregnancy out of fear it would harm her baby. Edwina gave birth to a beautiful baby girl, Ava, on January 20th 2005 and hoped to get back on LDN after she finished breastfeeding. Recently, I hooked up with Edwina on Facebook. Facebook is a fast growing internet web café. Edwina told me that she no longer takes LDN because she felt that it didn't help her enough. She decided that she can control her MS better with the best bet diet, plenty of rest and a good mental attitude. Everybody with MS or any autoimmune illness must be encouraged to treat themselves as they deem best because they know their bodies the best. I will always keep in touch with Edwina and wish her nothing but the very best.

Lorna and Terry relentlessly campaigned in Scotland and on April 12th 2004, The Herald newspaper in Glasgow, Scotland, carried a feature article: "MS Victim Finds Hope in Heroin Users' Drug; Campaign Launched for Urgent Trials of Naltrexone."

The article mentioned the increasing number of people who were petitioning for holding clinical trials specifically among people with MS in order that LDN could be licensed for their use, and detailed a success story. That was all thanks to Lorna's efforts. I was delighted that she managed to get her story in the paper because at the time, it was not an easy thing to do.

As a group, the LDN campaign team is relentless in their efforts and determination to get LDN to all those that

197

could benefit. Our priority is a large scale clinical trial. We are campaigning daily worldwide and when somebody finally takes the initiative to carry out a large scale scientific trial, it will be because of the daily efforts of all the alliances that have formed around the world as a result of LDN experience. I am very grateful for the many wonderful people I have met through LDN.

Chapter 29

"A happy family is but an earlier heaven."
Gerorge Bernard Shaw

efore I flew to Ireland in April 2004, I decided that I wanted to contact the Irish Government, but I knew that telling my story would not be good enough. I needed to be able to tell them exactly what I wanted them to do and figured out that I wanted them to do a clinical trial. They have everything to gain with the successful outcome of a trial so it made sense. I called Dr. Bihari and asked him if he would draw up a trial proposal for the Irish Government for LDN and MS that I could take to Ireland and present to them. As always, Dr. Bihari was more than willing to help. He agreed and thought it a sensible plan. The proposal wasn't ready before I flew so he agreed to fax it to me when I settled.

On April 23rd 2004, I flew to Ireland with my girls.

They loved to travel and were so easy to manage. They even had their own luggage that they packed themselves. They felt all grown up. The journey was fun. They were out of diapers, bottles and pacifiers, so compared to previous trips, it was relaxing. We arrived in Shannon and were greeted by Mom, Dad and Annie. As always, it was a fun visit.

The whole family gathered in Renmore in Mom and Dad's house. All of my brothers and their wives and children and my Aunt Kathleen were there. I met two new nephews, Ethan and James, and my first niece, Christina. Mom had a path worn out to the Poor Clares praying for her family to settle near her and was pleased that she succeeded in gathering all of her sons. My distance kept that path fresh.

It was wonderful to see everyone. Mom and Annie cooked a fantastic meal and when we were sitting around afterwards, Pat asked me what my plans were. I told them that I wanted to go on radio because I wanted to tell everyone about LDN. At first everyone laughed because they thought I was joking.

I assured them I wasn't and told them that I wanted them to help me. Among all of them and their friends somebody had to have some connection with a radio station, I thought. Then, my Aunt Kathleen rattled off a number, "double seven, double zero, double seven," she said.

Everyone looked at her and she repeated the number and said that I should call it first thing Monday morning and ask to speak with Keith Finnegan. We all cracked up laughing and teased her for knowing the number off by heart. Many comical references were made as to why she would know such a number until she confessed that she went on the show to point out the different petrol prices across the country. It bothered her and rightly that prices are not uniform.

Aunt Kathleen liked the way Keith handled the story and told me that he was very down to earth and a popular broadcaster. My brother Vince said that I should try Gerry Ryan, a popular national Irish radio presenter. He said that he found Gerry very helpful one Christmas when he needed a turkey recipe. I laughed at the thought of Vince cooking Gerry's turkey. Dad asked Mom and Annie if Vince hurt their feelings by asking Gerry for the recipe. He asked them a couple of times, but they never answered. After a comical discussion about radio, I decided that to want to go on radio to talk about LDN was perfectly normal. They all wished me luck with Keith who we agreed, in the end, was the most sensible target.

First thing Monday morning I called Galway Bay FM and asked to speak with Keith Finnegan. A lady named Fionnuala answered the phone and asked me for my story. She said that she was in charge of gathering potential stories and advised me to e-mail her immediately. She assured me that she would review it and pass it on to Keith if she thought that it would interest him. I logged on to Dad's computer and hammered out the story and appended Mom's cell phone number.

Then I hit the road with the children to head for Donegal. Mom and Annie followed me in a car behind. Before we reached Sligo, which is about two hours from Galway and half way to Donegal, Fionnuala called me on Mom's cell phone. She loved the story and said that they would run it without a problem. I couldn't believe it. She asked me if Brendan Quinn and Robert, whom I had mentioned in the story, would be willing to participate. She explained that they would make the story more plausible because Robert is actually on LDN and Brendan is the pharmacist preparing it in Galway. I assured her that they would oblige and told her that in order to make the show really credible we needed Dr. Bihari. She asked me if I thought he would be game. I was positive that he would play so I asked her to phone him and give it a shot.

I intended to phone Robert, Brendan and Dr. Bihari to let them know what I was doing but I lost my signal on the road so they all received a call out of the blue from Galway Bay FM. They figured out that I was behind it all pretty fast. Everybody was game and the show was scheduled for Friday April 30th at 11:10 a.m.. I called Dr. Bihari after everything was set and he assured me that he was delighted to participate.

After a wonderful visit with Noel's parents in Fahan, we headed to Arranmore Island to visit Grandpa Neilus. He looked wonderful. He still had a healthy glow about him and was still able to weld and work twelve hour days if he had to. His Parkinson's was in remission without question.

I love visiting Arranmore and catching up with people I grew up with. Angela is a good friend of mine and as we caught up I shared with her that I was pretty sure that I was pregnant. She thought it funny, as did I. She assumed that a potential pregnancy implied that Noel was doing well, which pleased her.

After a short visit on the Island, the children and I began our journey back to Galway on Thursday April 29th, with Mom and Annie a step behind. We all stopped in Letterkenny and I picked up a pregnancy test when Mom and Annie ran off shopping with the girls. That was a crazy day.

As only I would probably do, I took the test in a local pub, just because it was beside the pharmacy and I was in a rush to get back to the car to get on the road for Galway. The test was positive. I was pregnant. I laughed and called Noel. He was elated. He was so excited that he could hardly contain himself. He wished me luck for the radio show in the morning and told me that he would listen to it on the internet.

At that point, the radio show was the farthest thing from my mind and I headed to the car. I immediately told Mom and Annie that I was pregnant and they instantly started planning another trip to New Jersey for the birth. I think they were afraid to ask me how I found out, but I told them what I did. I made Annie laugh out loud and forced Mom to pretend that she didn't hear me. That happened a lot with us. They were both very happy with the unexpected news.

I can't help but think that maybe my brother Phil is correct in thinking that LDN boosts fertility considering Kate, Edwina and I all conceived quite quickly after starting LDN with very little effort.

Vince's wife Helen called me on the road to Galway to tell me that I have the longest pregnancies because I tell people so soon. She said that most people at least wait until the test dries before announcing. I laughed because it was true.

Chapter 30

"Even if you are a minority of one, the truth is the truth."
Mohandas Gandhi

D r. Bihari faxed me his proposal for an LDN trial in
Ireland for MS the next morning shortly before the
radio show. It was very interesting. Part of it read:

*"The autoimmune disease in which LDN is used most at
present is Multiple Sclerosis (MS). Dr. Bihari currently has
384 patients with MS in his medical care in a private practice setting in New York City. These patients have been on
LDN for an average of 2.5 years with a range of one week
to nineteen years. The overall results of treatment with this
drug have been excellent. Only three of the 384 patients
have shown any attacks. To be more specific, one of these
three, who started LDN eighteen years ago, at the age of
twenty-two in 1988, had one attack after five years on the
drug, thirty days after stopping it. The patient resumed*

LDN when the attack appeared and has had none in the thirteen years since. The second of the three, a forty-one-year-old woman, had an episode of optic neuritis which cleared in four weeks, after eighteen months on LDN. The last of the three was a patient who experienced an episode of numbness in the left leg after eight months on LDN, not previously present, which cleared after three weeks. The other 381 patients with MS have had no sign of disease activity since starting LDN."

It went on to state that there were, at that time, several thousand people with MS on LDN, who had their LDN prescribed by their physicians after reading about it on the LDN website. It then proposed a twelve month placebo controlled study of LDN at 3 mg. It recommended a sample size of 300 patients, 2/3's on the drug and 1/3 on placebo and estimated the cost to be less than 1 million Euro. That estimate did not account for MRIs, but it all sounded very reasonable and enticing.

Robert phoned me that morning to meet for coffee before the interview. I laughed when he congratulated me on my pregnancy because it reminded me of how fast news spreads in Galway. It was of course his sister-in-law and my friend, Coirle, who updated him. That was the first time I actually met Robert. I found him very relaxed and warm. We headed to the studio and I wasn't nervous at all because I didn't have time to think about it all week. Actually, I was so distracted for the week that I really didn't prepare so when I put on the headphones the nerves really hit me and I had to clear my throat a couple of times to combat them until I warmed up.

Overall the show went very well. I think that everybody I know in Ireland tuned in and the response was overwhelming. People all over the world tuned in because I posted on some LDN websites that Dr. Bihari was going to speak on the radio and they could hear it live from the Galway Bay FM website.

Robert gave a very relaxed and compelling personal account of his LDN experience and Brendan stated very clearly that he was sure that Dr. Bihari discovered something huge because he was seeing LDN work for people all over Ireland. Dr. Bihari explained LDN in terms that everyone could understand and relate to. His manner was confident, but laid back. He was in no way pushy, just matter of fact and sincere. He shared that he and Jacquie were taking LDN as a cancer preventative for twelve years and he listed all of the cancers that he believed LDN would effectively treat or prevent. Dr. Bihari listed a number of illnesses for which he also believed LDN held potential: Alzheimers, Rheumatoid Arthritis, Parkinson's, Sarcoidosis and Lupus. He assured people that after many years on the drug his bloodwork was normal. He was absolutely convinced and very convincing that LDN is a safe drug.

By all accounts the Keith Finnegan Show was a big success for LDN. Family members whom I had tried to explain the LDN theory to for a long time finally got it and wanted to try it. Actually, most of my school friends also finally understood and the word started to spread again like wildfire. I joked that the next time I want my family and friends to hear what I have to say I will have to call Keith. Soon after the show, I was quickly inundated with e-mail again and only too delighted to respond.

Lorna called Robert to say that she heard the show on the internet and told him that she thought that we did a fine job. That night I met up with a couple of school friends who could not believe that I didn't broadcast my pregnancy. We went out for dinner and laughed about the radio show. I told them that the funniest part of the whole thing was

Mom. She was reversing into the driveway in Renmore when she heard me on the car radio and rammed the car into the wall and took off the back bumper. I laughed when I saw it and assured Dad that I was positive it looked worse than it was. Things looking much worse than they actually were, was the type of common comfort cast in the Boyle household and guaranteed to aggravate.

A good friend of mine in Galway, Jane Whiriskey, is a nurse and called people she wanted to know about LDN. Another friend, Helen Diskin, said that she wanted to start LDN immediately for peace of mind. It was great. I have the best group of friends anybody could ever hope for.

I stated on the radio show that I was going to send the trial proposal to the Irish Government so I was keen to follow up on that. I didn't have time when I was in Ireland because by the time the Government offices opened that Monday I was due to fly back to New Jersey, and thank God I had no idea what lay ahead.

Chapter 31

"The highest calling in life is to be a soul friend."
                                                      St. Brigid

We flew into JFK Airport Monday May 3rd. Noel met us at the airport in his wheelchair and I was so glad to see him. We hate being apart. He was over the moon to see us, and the children climbed all over him talking in unison about their adventures in Ireland. Sara and Aisling resumed their normal positions; they sat on a knee each as he wheeled to the car. Annie held the handles of the chair and helped push all of them. They were a happy sight. That is how the four of them used to travel everywhere they went.

When the car was packed Noel hugged and kissed me. I was glad to be home. We hung outside the car in the rain to catch-up briefly. I told him that I felt great, the children were so good for the flight and we were going to have another memorable Christmas because the due date for the new baby was December 27th. Noel laughed and said that it would be our best Christmas ever.

Noel told me that I sounded great on the radio. Then he said that he managed to reseed our back yard on his own, when we were away. He clarified that he nearly broke his neck many times in the process, assured me that the neighbors must have thought that he was crazy and admitted that he was far too stubborn for his own good, but he swore that I would love it and think him brilliant. We joined the bedlam in the car and he drove us home.

After he put the children to bed, we made dinner and hung out for a while to catch-up properly. I was tired, so decided to take an early night. Things could not have been better.

Then, I woke at 2:00 a.m. with severe cramping and nausea and assumed that I was experiencing morning sickness because it was 7:00 a.m. in Ireland and I was most likely jetlagged. I thought little of it initially. I remembered Mom telling my sisters-in-law whenever they were brave enough to mention morning sickness, that they were very lucky, because morning sickness is the happiest sickness there is. It was commonly referred to as the "happy sickness" in the Boyle household.

By morning however, I feared something was wrong, so Noel took the day off work and I went to the doctor. The doctor told me to come back for a scan at 3:00 p.m.. A friend from the Moms Group, Stephanie Healy, took our children and Noel accompanied me for the afternoon appointment. Stephanie is a very close friend who will always drop everything to help me out. She is also a very useful friend and renowned for her cell phone habit. Whatever the catastrophe of the day is, she flips out her phone like a flick knife and organizes the troops.

By the time I got to the doctor's office I was very weak and probably dehydrated. I didn't have to wait long for medical attention because I passed out in their hallway. When I woke up, they did a scan and discovered that the pregnancy was ectopic and added that I needed immediate surgery because one of my tubes had burst and I was bleeding internally. I hated Noel being there for that. I so wished that he missed it, but there was no way that he would have. I will never forget the look on his face. I never saw a tear in his eye before, but I swear that I saw one that day. He got the fright of his life. For a second, he thought that I was going to die. He went from the happy expectant father to widower with three young girls in a split second and I felt dreadful for him. Then he snapped out of it and took control and brought me to the hospital. I think that he was fine as long as there was something for him to do, but once the doctors took over and hooked me up to everything I saw that look of fear return to his face. Thank God another friend of ours, Kristen Peterson, worked in the hospital. She came over to me and I told her that I was fine because I genuinely thought that I was, and asked her to make sure that Noel was okay. I wanted her to take care of Noel. She was wonderful. I will always remember her for being there.

When my blood pressure started to drop I asked the doctor to explain the situation to me. It was incredibly painful. The doctor told me that the situation was serious, and that they were trying to rush me into surgery as quickly as possible. He said that he didn't really know what to expect when they opened me up and then took the liberty of explaining to me that ectopic pregnancy is the leading cause of death from pregnancy in the U.S.. I actually laughed when he said that and told him quietly that my brother was a doctor in Ireland, and had a book with a chapter about good bedside manners that might be worth a read in his spare time. The nurse heard me and burst out laughing. I told Noel that there was a bright side. He could always write another witness speech for Cornerstone because this material was perfect. I was quite the comedienne.

When they were wheeling me in for surgery I didn't know if I would wake up again. I realized that I had no control and I accepted that. I was positive that if my number was up then it was simply up and there was nothing I could do about it. I was surprisingly calm. I firmly believed that God would look after Noel and my children if I couldn't. I was, however, greatly relieved when I woke up after the surgery and informed that it all went well. They tied the tube that burst and I could go home the following day.

I was familiar enough with MS to know that she would not let recent events fade easily. I knew she would rear her ugly head as a result of the stress Noel experienced and I knew that LDN was about to be put to the ultimate test. I was on guard for the monster to attack.

I was glad to get home to be with Noel and the children. I was also anxious to check my e-mail as I knew I had a lot of correspondence to catch up on from Ireland with regard to LDN. I was also eager to write to Rosemary. I was in constant e-mail contact with her, even from Ireland. I appreciated her support and wanted to let her that know everything was okay.

My e-mail correspondence with Rosemary always helped me figure things out and put things in perspective. I never knew e-mail could be such fun. My daughter, Annie Kate was still in her class so had filled her in somewhat, but I wanted to fill in the blanks. I told her that I was going to send the proposal to the Irish Government as soon as I could and she suggested that I should learn how to crochet or needlepoint. As always, Rosemary remained balanced, neutral and light with a little affection. I knew that she was relieved I was okay. It is only now as I review our correspondence do I see how focused on LDN I really was for quite a period. I also realize that Rosemary helped me more than she will ever know.

I predicted an MS attack in an e-mail to Rosemary before it happened. That was not by any means fortunetelling. It was simply familiarity with the beast.

Chapter 32

"Patience is the companion of wisdom"

St. Augustine

Shortly after my miscarriage, I started to research the Irish Government. I found a website with a list of every TD (member of Parliament of the Republic of Ireland) and their e-mail address. On May 14th 2004, I sent Dr. Bihari's trial proposal for LDN and MS direct to the Taoiseach Bertie AHern. I also sent a copy to the Minister for Finance, Charlie McCreevy and the Minister for Health at the time, Micheal Martin. Micheal D Higgins also received a copy because he used to lecture me in UCG. I also sent the proposal to various regional health boards who told me that it needed to be reviewed by Mr. Martin, the then Minister for Health. On May 19th I received the following e-mail from the Irish Government:

Mary Boyle Bradley

Dear Ms Bradley

I wish to acknowledge receipt of your e-mail dated 14 May 2004 which will be brought to the Taoiseach's attention as soon as possible.

Yours sincerely,

Michael
Taoiseach's Private Office

I didn't get excited because I knew that an acknowledgment meant very little after dealing with the South African Government. It is just a courtesy.

On May 18th Edwina and Robert managed to get the LDN story into the Irish Times. I sent that article as a follow-up to the same cross section of the Irish Government. I received an e-mail from everyone except Mr. Martin. They all said that it was Mr. Martin's job to review it and assured me that they forwarded him the information. My favorite reply came on June 11th. It read:

Dear Ms Bradley

The Taoiseach Mr. Bertie Ahern T.D. has asked me to refer to your e-mail of 9 June 2004 regarding your proposals concerning Multiple Sclerosis.

The Taoiseach has forwarded your correspondence to his colleague Mr. Micheál Martin T.D., Minister for Health and Children for his attention. He has asked the Minister to have the points you raised addressed and to respond directly to you.

The Taoiseach has asked me to extend his best wishes to you.

Yours sincerely,
Nick Reddy
Assistant Private Secretary to the Taoiseach

It was a nice birthday present to have Bertie wish me well.

It is January 2009 now. Mr. Martin never responded. Mary Harney is the current Irish Minster for Health and also never responded. Like I said, things take a great deal longer than I would like, but I have by no means given up.

The ideal ending for this story, of course, would be that the Irish or any Government decided to start a large scale LDN trial for MS and LDN, but a true story rarely ends ideally. The struggle continues and the snowball gets bigger everyday. A large scale trial will happen though. It will happen somewhere, someday. I do not doubt that for a second.

I know that many people don't have the luxury of time to wait for a large scale clinical trial, so I hope that my story will help someone, somewhere, stop their disease in the nick of time. I don't want anyone to leave it as long as we did. What if Noel found LDN when he was first diagnosed and his MS was invisible? Such thinking is too negative to dwell on. Such thinking could land me in a nuthouse. For justice and sanity, perhaps, I want to make sure that other people who are diagnosed with MS know that they can change their future. I believe with my heart and soul that people with MS can change their future for the better with LDN.

Chapter 33

"Life is not about surviving the storm.
We must learn how to dance in the rain."
Anonymous

Noel and I both felt a deep sense of loss after the miscarriage but an equally strong sense of gratitude for all that we had. We felt very fortunate to have three beautiful, healthy girls and each other, so we privately named the baby we lost and moved on. At first things seemed fine and I started to wonder if I needed to be on guard for another MS attack. Being an optimist, I thought that maybe LDN would work better than Dr. Bihari thought it would. Then I was reminded that sometimes that light I see at the end of a tunnel, is in fact an oncoming train. Noel started to relapse. He experienced his first relapse since he started LDN.

Part of me was definitely mentally prepared for Noel to

slip after the stress he experienced because when it happened I was not overly concerned about it. I was following people on the internet, in particular Goodshape's wife Polly. I knew that Polly slipped on occasion under stress or infection, but she always managed to bounce back given time. I was very sorry to hear that on May 7, 2004 Polly died from heart failure at age sixty-five. Heart conditions ran in her family, but she lived ten years longer than the average member of her immediate family. Her MS had been stable for four years on LDN and they were planning one more cruise that will never happen. Fritz Bell and Polly were married for forty-two years and many felt his grief. Since Polly died, Fritz changed his website to focus more on LDN instead of histamine, because he firmly believed that LDN is a miracle drug.

Reading about a relapse and watching one are two completely different things. I can only imagine what it must have felt like for Noel to physically endure another blow. We were so spoilt for so long, it was easy to believe, at times, that relapses would be a thing of the past now that we found LDN.

For the first time ever, Noel got angry with his MS, and rightly or wrongly I got caught in the crossfire. Nobody was more convinced than me that we were going to live happily ever after and although Noel did all in his power to remain mentally prepared for a relapse, my constant optimism wore him down and he let his guard down. Noel was not mentally prepared to relapse. He got angry.

Then he got angry for getting angry. He hated not handling his decline with grace. He really had to readjust his focus until he found a way of dealing once again with an MS relapse. I cannot express how awful I felt. I knew that in many ways, I was responsible for his mental state.

My concerns went way beyond Noel very fast. I realized almost immediately that I had raised the hopes of many, many people who were more than likely, in the course of their life, going to experience sufficient stress or illness that would most likely cause them to slip. To slip when you are convinced that you won't makes that slip much, much worse. It was a dreadful feeling and it hit home very hard that a level of responsibility is essential when dishing out medical advice without training on various websites. I always tried to qualify my advice with a note about my lack of medical training, but I now realized that that was not good enough. I realized that I don't know the whole LDN story or have all the answers. Without a clinical trial nobody does.

There are so many desperate people in desperate situations who really need LDN, but to reach the masses the right way it needs the backing of the medical community. I figured the only way to do all of the people justice and to maximize my time and efforts, was to fully dedicate my spare time to efforts for a clinical trial. That way everyone could embark on their personal LDN journey, with their eyes wide open, and the backing of the medical community to help them out in times of stress or infection. I want all the cards on the table for everyone to see, without illusion or false hope. That can only happen via a large scale clinical trial of LDN.

It was around that time, in July 2004, that I decided to write everything down in a series of e-mails to Rosemary and I have to confess that the experience has been cathartic and therapeutic.

To describe Noel's relapse, it was obvious that compared to the whopper of 1998, the 2004 one was very mild. Dr. Bihari called it a pseudo relapse because Noel did not experience any new symptoms. He experienced a reoccurrence of old symptoms with an exaggerated vengeance. His upper body remained very strong and thank God the relapse only affected his legs. Noel never reached his worst point pre LDN. He always remained better than he was before he started LDN.

Dr. Bihari prescribed steroids for Noel and they worked a little for a short while. Noel remained on 4.5 mg LDN while he took the steroids because Dr. Bihari believed that although on paper they work against each other, in his practice he found that it is not that straightforward. Steroids and LDN actually complement each other in times of relapse. Noel also took the DL Phenylalanine supplement and felt that it helped him a little initially, but not enough to keep taking it daily. I once again contemplated a walker for the house, but Noel asked me to wait for a while.

It is January 2009 now and Noel and I have ridden many waves since he first started taking LDN. Overall, Noel has lost some of what he initially gained from LDN, but his MS remains confined to his legs and bladder. He has not experienced any brand-new symptoms since he started taking LDN in September 2002. His MS is no longer creeping up his body. In many respects, we feel like we are living with an injury as opposed to a progressive degenerative disease.

I wish we found LDN sooner. I wish we found it when Noel's legs worked properly. I hate MS. I can see the good that it has brought to my family, but I still hate it and have no problem sharing that. Noel, on the other hand, feels honored in some respect, to help Jesus carry His cross and doesn't like it when I think negatively. Noel never, ever complains about having MS or asks for the chalice to be taken away. He believes that his MS is all part of God's plan for him. He gets angry now and then because his MS can be frustrating, but overall, I envy his faith. I think that Noel gets angry because he knows that he has many, many years of living left with MS to pass the test of life and be with Jesus. He knows that the progression has stopped. In some respects, it was easier for him to be a superhero when he was progressing rapidly and he believed that he didn't have long to live to pass the test. A short test of life can be easier than a long one. God, however, has certainly granted Noel every grace he needs to live with MS and Noel will always be my superhero.

Our three children have no hang-ups as a result of MS. If anything, MS has made them better people. Noel is always very honest with his daughters. He tells them all the time to think only of what they can do and to never focus on what they can't. And he makes sure that we never miss Sunday mass. Noel is a wonderful husband and father and I know for a fact that I could not love or respect anybody more than I do him.

Noel has to exercise rigorously to maintain muscles in his legs that he no longer uses. When he walks, he doesn't use the muscles typically used for walking and so, over time, he has lost some muscle mass. We have noticed that if he exercises and cuts out refined sugars and processed foods, he walks a great deal better. But, Noel also works fifty hours a week (if you count his commute), so it is not easy for him to exercise as much as he would like. The company we started to work for when we graduated from university, Wilco, was sold to ADP and then the division that Noel worked in, was spun off to become Broadridge, so Noel does something with computers and finance with Broadridge in Jersey City. He explained his job to me many times, but I still don't fully get it. The stock market baffles me. We are thankful that he is no longer a barman, because he wouldn't be able to work. That said, he can still make a good drink and now and then we break his diet, but he pays dearly when he drinks alcohol.

Noel may not look like a poster child for LDN because his mobility is greatly affected, but I think that he is the perfect poster child because LDN does not cure MS. LDN stops MS from progressing. There are many LDN success stories on the internet. Google LDN. From Facebook to YouTube, every site has an LDN community. Some people take LDN and get out of wheelchairs. Although I am happy for such folk and, believe me, nobody is happier than I for their success and I love them all, I must stress that it is very dangerous to take LDN and think that it will reverse MS. It might reverse some symptoms. It might reverse them for a short period or for forever even. Whatever symptoms it reverses, for however long, is a bonus. The promise is that LDN stops progression. Noel has not experienced a worse day post LDN than pre LDN. That does not mean that he doesn't have bad days. He does. And under stress, MS will still attack with a vengeance, but we are beating the odds and living as happily ever after as possible thanks to LDN. I do wish we found it sooner though, like Robert and Paula, but thank God we found it when we did. Like I said, we found LDN in the nick of time.

Noel is, without question, better than he was pre LDN. This is the bottom line: despite the stresses life throws, after more than five years, Noel is still much better than he was pre LDN. He looks wonderful. All of his bloodwork is perfect. His doctor even told him that apart from having MS, Noel is in perfect health. I bet that he will outlive most of his peers thanks to LDN. He uses one or two canes to get around and relies on his wheelchair when he has errands to run, but he still walks all around the house, to and from his car and from his car to his work. He is still living a totally independent life and our married life could not be any better. I know that we are incredibly fortunate because I know two people who died from Primary Progressive MS. That is how serious

MS can get and I am under no illusion about that.

LDN is the best treatment for MS currently available. So far, it has given us five more wonderful years that we would not have enjoyed otherwise. We can live very happily with our current hand.

On the Parkinson's front, my Uncle Neilus continues to work twelve hour days in the shipyards. His Parkinson's, however, has progressed slightly despite LDN. He got a couple of great years out of LDN and continues to take LDN for his overall health, but his shake has spread a little. In December 2008, I accompanied Neilus to a neurologist appointment in New York City. I wanted to learn about all of the latest conventional PD therapies and see if there was anything Neilus could take to improve his quality of life because writing, shaving and welding had become increasingly difficult over the years. As expected, the top neurologist for PD in New York City had never heard of LDN, but said that he was surprised that my uncle had PD for so long and had progressed so slowly. He did not credit LDN. He said that Neilus was one of the lucky few. He told us that stem cell therapy for PD was at least ten years away from being a realistic option and that Neilus was at least ten years away from needing to consider any type of surgery. He started Neilus on one half tablet of Parcopa 25mg/100mg twice daily. That dose is even lower than the recommended lowest possible dose of the medication. He chose Parcopa because Neilus has a sensitive stomach when it comes to medicine and Parcopa bypasses the stomach. It dissolves in the mouth and gets to work right away. I am not, by any means, anti conventional medicine as long as it works. Please God Parcopa will help his shake which is the only symptom he has that affects his quality of life. Neilus will not stop LDN because I firmly believe it is helping him. I also learned that my uncle used to go off

LDN for a week here and there over the years. I begged him not to do that ever again.

I also accompanied my uncle to his annual physical in December 2008. His doctor told him that all of his blood work was absolutely perfect. Apart from having PD, Neilus is in perfect shape. The last time I spoke with Dr. Bihari about LDN and Parkinson's, he told me that although some of his other PD patients also progressed over time, others did not, and he added that their overall health was much better on LDN. I still recommend LDN to everybody I know with PD. The most passionate advocate for LDN and PD is a friend of mine named Destiny Ellen. She believes that LDN has proven to be a wonder drug for her father, Bentley, who has PD. She wants everyone with PD to know about LDN.

On the cancer front, Dr. Bihari reports that more than 60% of patients with cancer may significantly benefit from LDN treatment. I also believe that LDN makes many existing cancer therapies more effective. LDN definitely helps kill many cancers. I have met people with cancer on LDN who are living happily ever after. Sadly, Mom did not fall into that category. In January 2005, my family discovered that her breast cancer had spread to her bones despite LDN. Since then, we tried absolutely everything to save Mom, but she died on August 6th 2007. No medicine, not even LDN will keep any of us alive forever. No matter how long we live, we are all just passing through and when my time comes to pass I am grateful that my mother taught me how to die right. There is no finer lesson in life.

On November 29th, 2008, my sister-in-law, Evana (Phil's wife), gave birth to a beautiful baby girl and named her Maureen Teresa Boyle after our mother. I am eternally grateful to Evana for such a loving gesture and tribute to Mom.

There are few things I know for certain, but I know for a fact that no two people ever lived who loved each other more than Mom and I. Thank God, I have been blessed with a sense of her presence daily and amazingly, am coping very well. Mom never left me and I don't think that she ever will. We are too comfortable together. I wrote her story down and will publish it as soon as I can. I called it *"Going Nowhere."* We learned a heck of a lot about cancer during Mom's final year. Cancer is an even bigger business than MS. I know that my mother died and is a poor poster child for what we discovered, but I believe we found the answer for cancer sufferers. Too late for Mom, but in the nick of time for others. Friends of mine are proving the theory today, but that is a whole other story.

Noel and I remain happily settled in New Jersey and have no intention of moving in the near future because it has become our home and the town, our family. We are delighted to be part of such a caring community. We love the town, schools and church. Thank God we have a wonderful quality of life.

Today, there is a fast growing worldwide grassroots movement working towards the scientific recognition of LDN. As more people experience the effects of the drug, the stronger this movement becomes. It is impossible to search the internet now for MS information without finding something on LDN. There are numerous LDN websites in many different languages. People are screaming for their success stories to be heard. There are also numerous news clippings from all around the world, begging for a large scale clinical trial.

My plea to every reader is that they Google LDN. Visit the official LDN website at www.ldninfo.org to find out all of the latest news regarding clinical trials and upcoming events. There are many. There is more than enough published scien-

tific data there to convince any doctor to prescribe LDN
thanks in part to the efforts of Dr. Jill Smith from Penn State
and her clinical trial of LDN for Crohn's disease and Dr. Gi-
roni's pilot trial of LDN for Primary Progressive MS. I will
append a list of my favorite LDN websites to this book and
my contact details so that we can keep in touch. My own
website is www.marybradleybooks.com. Noel designed it for
me and I think he did a fine job.

Where is Dr. Bihari? Dr. Bernard Bihari is living in
New York City with his wife, Jacquie. He is in his late sev-
enties and all but retired from his practice due to ill health
(he is still able to do an occasional telephone consultation).
A few years ago, Dr. Bihari fell down a flight of stairs in
the Waldorf Hotel and broke his arm. Since then, he frac-
tured his hip and then his neck, and has been in and out of
physical rehab institutions and developed seizures. I hope
and pray for his daily comfort. He continues to take LDN.

Just how right is Dr. Bihari? I believe that he discovered something as important as penicillin. And safe enough
that it could become part of a nightly multivitamin in the
future. LDN works for such an array of illnesses, it stands
to reason that it will complement many therapies in the future by boosting our immune systems. I am eternally thankful that Dr. Bihari crossed my path.

The internet has proved to be a remarkable tool for
LDN community building. The people are passionate and
dedicated so I have no doubt that LDN will hit the masses.
The question is not *if* LDN will be scientifically recognized, but rather when and by whom. The issue is not
whether or not LDN works, but rather how well does it
work. And I don't doubt that many lives will benefit from
the use of LDN in the future, but I cannot help but wonder
exactly how many.

LDN websites worth visiting

www.ldninfo.org
www.marybradleybooks.com
www.skipspharmacy.com/
www.ldnresearchtrust.org/
www.ldners.org
http://video.google.com/videoplay?docid=8313092875696
096715
http://www.thepetitionsite.com/1/sign-support-the-
campaign-for-research-trials-in-low-dose-naltrexone-
for-multiple-sclerosis
www.ldn.proboards3.com/
www.goodshape.net/

A Remedy for Anxiety from my brother, Dr. Phil Boyle, that helped me:

MATHEW 6; 25-34

Therefore I tell you, do not worry about your life, what you will eat or drink; or about your body, what you will wear. Is not life more important than food, and the body more important than clothes? Look at the birds of the air; they do not sow or reap or store away in barns, and yet your heavenly Father feeds them. Are you not much more valuable than they? Who of you by worrying can add a single hour to his life? And why do you worry about clothes? See how the lilies of the field grow. They do not labor or spin. Yet I tell you that not even Solomon in all his splendor was dressed like one of these. If that is how God clothes the grass of the field, which is here today and tomorrow is thrown into the fire, will he not much more clothe you, O you of little faith? So do not worry, saying, "What shall we eat?" or "What shall we drink?" or "What shall we wear?" For the pagans run after all these things, and your heavenly Father knows that you need them. But seek first his kingdom and his righteousness, and all these things will be given to you as well. Therefore do not worry about tomorrow, for tomorrow will worry about itself. Each day has enough trouble of its own.

CPSIA information can be obtained at www.ICGtesting.com
Printed in the USA
BVOW03s1717041113

335353BV00001B/23/P